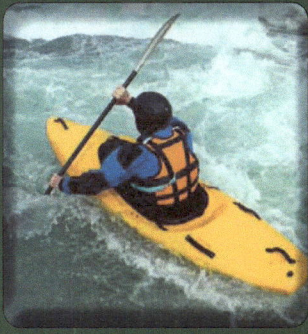

4 SEASON FITNESS

GRANT HILDERBRAND, PH.D.

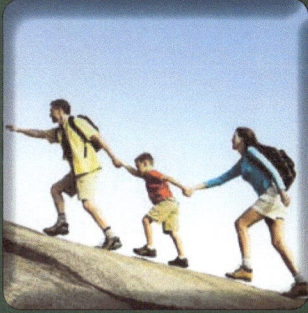

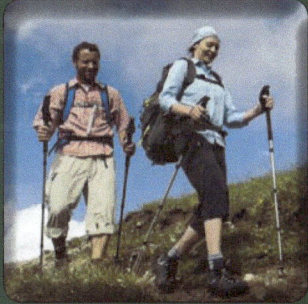

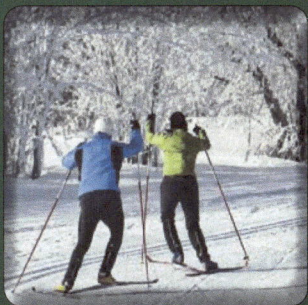

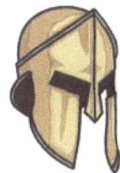

SPARTAN FITNESS ALASKA
ANCHORAGE, ALASKA

WWW.SPARTANFITNESSALASKA.COM

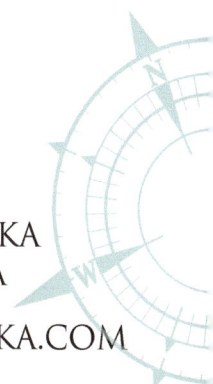

Published by
Spartan Fitness Press

The Publication Arm of
Spartan Fitness Alaska, LLC
5800 Kalgin Drive
Anchorage, AK 99516
www.spartanfitnessalaska.com

4 Season Fitness: A Practical Guide to the Lifetime Enjoyment of
the Great Outdoors

Design by Adrienne Wilkerson © January 2010
Beacon Publishing & Design, LLC. www.beacon-design.com

Copy Editing by Jane Mackay, Janemac Editing
www.janemac.net

ISBN 13: 978-0-9841784-0-7
ISBN 10: 0-98-417840-6

TABLE OF CONTENTS

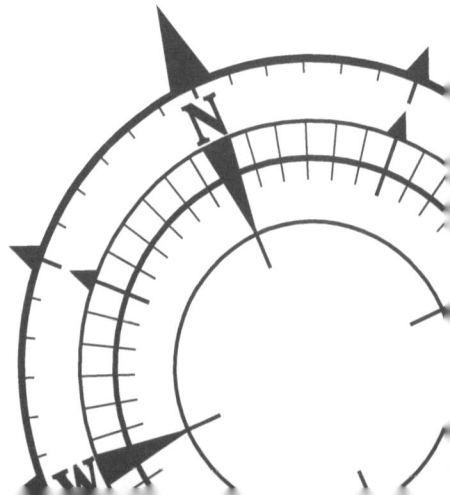

ACKNOWLEDGEMENTS

At its heart, this book is about relationships. The journey that started with the conception of an idea and ended with the book held in your hands is the product of relationships. This book was born of the efforts of a community of friends and this collective collaboration is what I am most proud of and most inspired by.

Specifically, I want to thank Ross Russo who provided insightful comments and suggestions on early drafts of this manuscript. Prior to that, Ross helped the idea take shape while serving as the consummate hiking partner. Howard Golden is a long-time friend and colleague and his review greatly improved organization and flow. Pat Fedrick offered her time as a reviewer, support for the spirit of this project, and some of the best hugs in the world for my family and me. Harlow Robinson provided some very good editorial suggestions that resulted in a more readable manuscript. As important, Harlow shares my belief in the link between time in the outdoors and our holistic well being. His support for this book further inspired me. I'm honored to have our kids growing up together. Taughnee Stone of Endeavor Creative offered unending enthusiasm for the project and belief in my approach to developing a functional, lifelong fitness. Adrienne Wilkerson of Beacon Publishing & Design crafted a vision that perfectly captured the essence of the message I was striving to convey. Jane Mackay of Janemac Editing provided professional proof reading and some light copy editing of the text. Without question, this book is better for her diligence and keen eye.

The exercise photos are key to bringing the words to life and Katia Pronzati, Zoey Hilderbrand, and Taughnee Stone did a wonderful job of visually directing and capturing the actions and movements. I am also indebted to the Anchorage fitness community, especially Polaris Athletic Club (Bill Frick), and Powerhouse Gym (Joy Shankar) for their support.

My kids, Devon, Zoey, Jonah, and Mila, are my purest motivation as they make me want to stay young forever. Finally, thank you to Katia Pronzati, my wife and my best friend, for her inspiration, faith, and companionship. She has simultaneously broadened my horizons and brought warmth to my world.

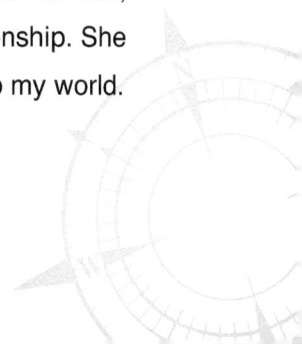

INTRODUCTION

"LIFE DOESN'T HAPPEN IN A STRAIGHT LINE"

When I received word of my grandfather's death, I was catching and radio-collaring grizzly bears in Denali National Park, the heart of the Alaska Range and home to the continent's highest peak. Each week I would walk two miles from my small camper to the pay phone at a nearby lodge. By chance, I reached my mom the morning after he passed. I idolized my grandfather as if he were the north on my compass. Though he had been ill for some time, I wasn't prepared for his passing. I just couldn't reconcile the reality that a man, so much larger than life to me, was mortal.

The logistics of leaving the Park and the schedules for flights departing Fairbanks dictated that I stay in Denali for an additional day before beginning the pilgrimage home. Thus, my colleagues and I continued our work. Three hours after getting the somber news, I found myself sitting atop a ridge on the north side of Mt. McKinley, just east of the Muldrow glacier. We had darted the first bear of the day and I had stayed behind to ensure her safe awakening from the anesthesia, while the helicopter and other staff had moved on to continue the day's work and handle additional bears. I was left alone to ponder my grandfather's passing surrounded by the fall colors of the arctic tundra and the cold breeze coming off the glacier at the foot of the granite massif that was Denali. Somehow, feeling so small next to the grandeur of this place made my loss easier to take, a natural occurrence, a part of processes eons old.

I have always felt most at home in nature. Many of my fondest childhood memories take me back to my family's farm in central Missouri. In the northern Ozarks the passing of time was marked by the fresh smell of dew on spring mornings, the feel of the perpetual dust from working the hay clinging to my skin in the summer heat, the crunching sound of frosted fall leaves underfoot, and the chilled look of dormant trees bristling in winter winds. Fishing in the creeks and ponds, catching bullfrogs and fireflies, seeing the first fawns of the year, and exploring the woods provided me endless adven-

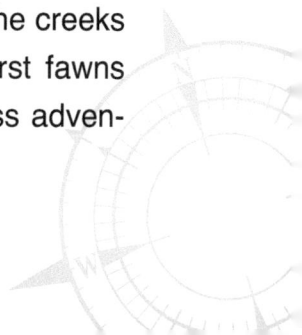

tures and fueled my curiosity. My home wasn't defined by walls and doors and windows, it was a sense of place. The lessons I learned at my grandfather's heels were seldom spoken, just demonstrated. At eighty years old, he could still stack square hay bales all day long, pull a calf when the cow's efforts failed, and walk ten miles cross-country, hardly breaking a sweat.

I eventually found my way to a career that allowed me to earn a living working largely outdoors. My office had no door or windows. They weren't required. Working as a wildlife biologist in Alaska, I saw something new, something truly amazing nearly every day. For reasons necessary if not good, I accepted promotions, took on more and more responsibility, and found myself farther and farther from the field. In time, I lost my sense of place.

I was going through a rough patch (to put it mildly) in my personal life. I was grappling with divorce, death, and loss. The processes of grief, accountability, self-assessment, and forgiveness led to significant growth and new-found hope. The challenges I faced led to re-evaluation of many aspects of my life: my relationships, my career, my dreams, my responsibilities, and my passions. I decided I had a lot to learn, a lot to give, and a lot to receive. It was time to plot a new path.

I wove together my love for wild places, my thirst for learning, and my desire for meaningful relationships by founding a personal training and fitness consulting business in Anchorage, Alaska. It has evolved into one of the most rewarding endeavors of my life.

Paramount is the intimacy of the relationships I develop with my clients. Clients share their aspirations, their fears, their insecurities, and their hopes for the future. As a trainer, I am allowed to act as a guide and witness the sense of personal growth and achievement earned by my clients. My approach to fitness focuses on functionality, transcending the walls that separate us from the world outside. I strive to address the trinity of emotional well-being, physical health, and our sense of place in the natural world. This book is an extension of my commitment, my advocacy for nature and its importance to our quality of life.

Life doesn't happen in a straight line. If you train for a predictable world, you will be ill-prepared. This book will provide you with a path leading to a foundation of broad and practical fitness that will translate effectively into daily life and the widest spectrum of outdoor recreational activities; a fitness without walls.

At its core, this book is about relationships: your relationship with yourself and your body, your relationship with the natural world, and your relationships with those who matter most to you. My hope is that this guide will provide you with the confidence and physical skills you need to help you get out to enjoy and embrace the world outside your door and to be able to share this sense of place with your friends, your spouse, your kids, and your grandkids. Here is to you and to your memories yet to be made.

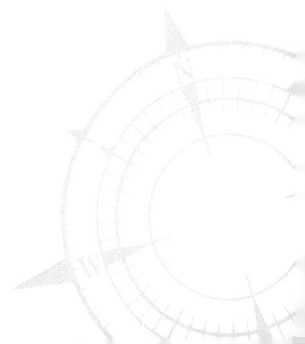

*"I WANT TO DO
AS MUCH AS I CAN,
AS WELL AS I CAN,
FOR AS LONG AS I CAN"*

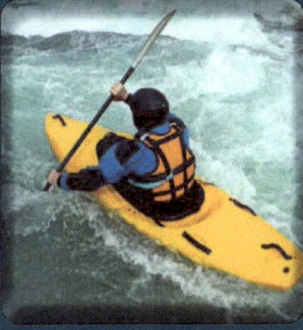

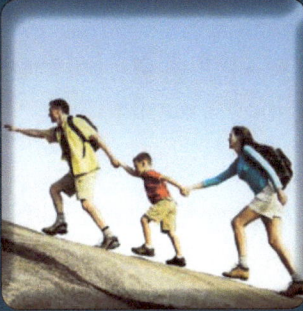

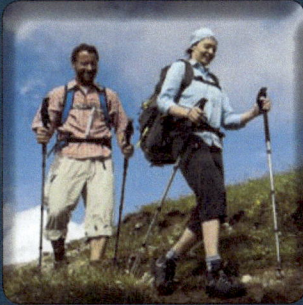

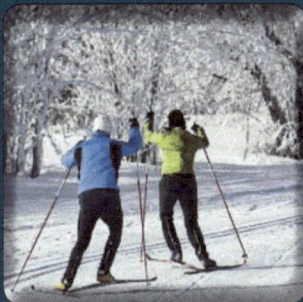

CHAPTER 1:
FITNESS & THE
OUTDOOR RECREATION
GENERALIST

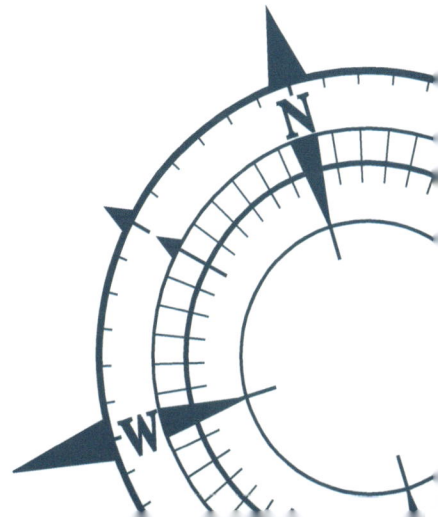

I'm not world class at anything. I never have been and never will be. Most of us aren't. I'm also not a specialist. If anything, I'm the opposite. Over the past year, I have hiked, climbed, run, biked, kayaked, canoed, tide-pooled, snorkeled, downhill skied, skate-skied, hunted, fished, and chopped wood. I didn't do it for ribbons or medals. I engaged in these activities simply because I enjoy them. More to the point, I enjoy sharing these experiences with others. I choose to live in a magnificent part of the world, one blessed with four distinct seasons and an endless variety of options for those who love recreating in the outdoors. I'm not world class at anything, but I strive for competency at a wide variety of physical activities. I want to do as much as I can, as well as I can, for as long as I can.

My view of fitness has evolved through time. I worked out with weights and on "cardio" machines throughout high school to improve my performance in various sports, and power-lifted competitively and successfully through college. After graduation, I continued the same basic training regimen through my twenties. In my early thirties, I could bench press about 400 lbs, squat about 600lbs, and run a six minute mile. I was "gym fit."

Then, about five years ago came a seminal moment. I started dating Katia, an amazing woman who has since become my wife, the adoptive mother of my daughter, and mother to my son and soon-to-arrive baby girl. She grew up in Italy, at the base of the Alps and, to this day, lives for the outdoors. Skiing, hiking, and berry picking top her list of favorite things, especially if accompanied by her

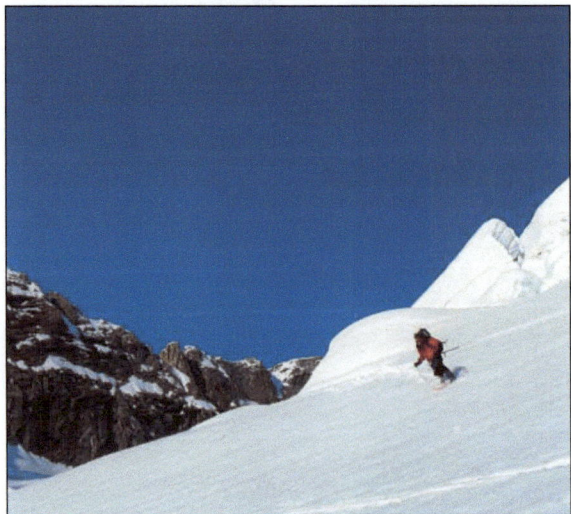

dog, Echo. As we started spending more and more time together and venturing into the wilderness on various outings, it became apparent to me that she could outperform me at nearly every physical activity we engaged in. It was all quite humbling. Further, I was becoming more and more cognizant of my mortality and my responsibility as a father. My time horizon expanded as I became more focused on my future quality of life and physical capacities at age fifty, sixty, seventy, eighty, and beyond.

The realization came to me that, despite spending significant time and effort in the gym, when I ventured out of the air-conditioning and off the pavement, I was ill-prepared. I was slow, clumsy, and easily winded. Further, I lacked the confidence, and thus the willingness to try new things. After coming to terms with this reality, I accepted that I had aged a bit and that my eating habits needed to improve. All told, my fitness regimen poorly served the changing desires and priorities of the life I was choosing to live.

I wanted to be healthy. I wanted to be proficient. Most of all, I wanted to remain active and share experiences with those who mattered most to me. In essence, I wanted to someday be the man to my grandchildren that my grandfather was to me. Through a lot of research, experimentation, observation, professional education, and hard work, I largely retooled my tool box. I refined my approach and enhanced the efficiency and functionality of my training. I removed the distinction between the worlds inside and outside the gym. The approach that has served me well is the same approach I now utilize successfully with my clients.

There is something both primal and serene about connecting with and being one with nature. Our attraction to the world outside our door is innate, as unavoidable

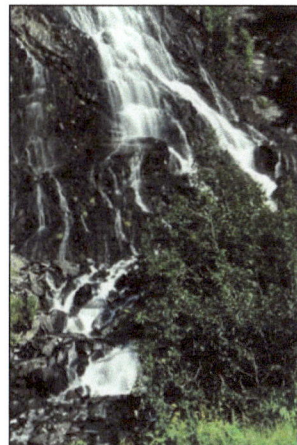

as the tides. It is a sense of place shared by both young and old. My three-year-old son constantly bangs on our porch door, wailing "outside, outside" in protest when confined to our house for inconveniences such as baths or meals. In the same spirit, I've had friends and family who, when facing death, asked that their remains be scattered to a favored mountain, stream, or vista.

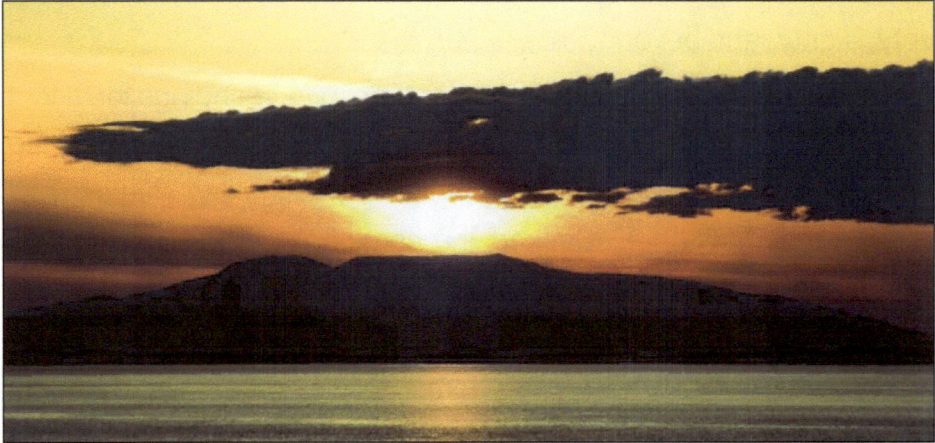

By nature, we are a community of outdoor recreation generalists. Our level of physical fitness is the foundation of our individual competency across a wide spectrum of activities. Our fitness is both dynamic and organic. It changes through time and can be shaped and honed. Left unattended, it can deteriorate; however, tended to appropriately, it can be improved and refined at any age.

Traditionally, fitness texts and programs have focused on one of several aspects of general fitness or outcomes of varied exercise regimes. Much attention has been paid to the roles of exercise and diet, and their implications for weight loss for aesthetic purposes. The medical community and exercise physiology researchers have long understood the wide-ranging health benefits of exercise such as improved cardiac function through aerobic training and increased bone density resulting from resistance training. Many efforts have focused on the development of the perfect physique and largely emphasize diet and weight training (i.e., body building). Sports-specific training can hone an athlete's ability to thrive in specific events or sports and, due to the social import of organized sport, significant ink has been dedicated to improving athletic performance.

I favor a broader concept of fitness, one that acknowledges the importance of cardiovascular and muscular endurance (aerobic capacity), power (anaerobic capacity), range of motion, as well as agility and balance. Most importantly, it acknowledges that these fitness categories form an overall mosaic and attention must be paid to each component. I further argue that the most functional and efficient way to train is to blur the lines between the different categories. Time spent in the gym is beneficial to functional capacity as it allows us to fully and efficiently develop all components of our overall fitness; however, we are striving for a fitness that matters not only in the gym, but in daily life when you load the groceries, pick up your child or grandchild, or empty the dishwasher and put away the plates on an upper shelf. Further, we are looking for capacities and abilities that translate to the slope, the trail, or the water; thus, fitness can't be assessed solely by your body fat percentage, single lift bench press weight, or 5 km time. Functional fitness has to account for your ability to participate and succeed in daily life and in the activities you enjoy. It has to account for quality of life.

An additional important and often underappreciated aspect of fitness lies between your ears. There are specific neurochemical responses to exercise that provide significant health benefits and these are not to be discounted. But what I am more interested in is the relationship that individuals develop with their body as they train.

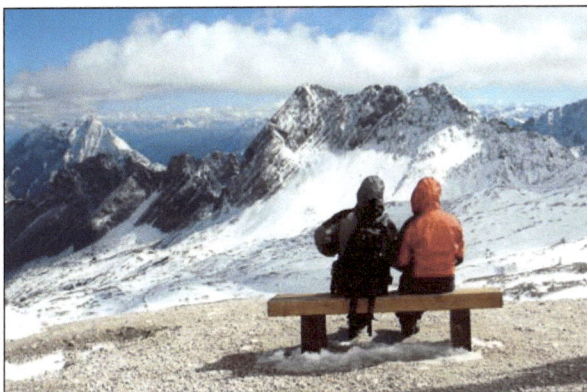

An innate, but often underdeveloped and long-forgotten kinesthetic awareness evolves, meaning trained individuals accurately sense the location and position of their body in space. They also have an acute sense of their physical capacities and the result is an increased confidence in their ability to try and succeed at new and challenging tasks in daily life and recreation. The link between improved functional fitness and increased "confidence capacity" is where one's life truly improves, where the horizon expands, where limits become benchmarks to be surpassed. These are the fruits of our labor.

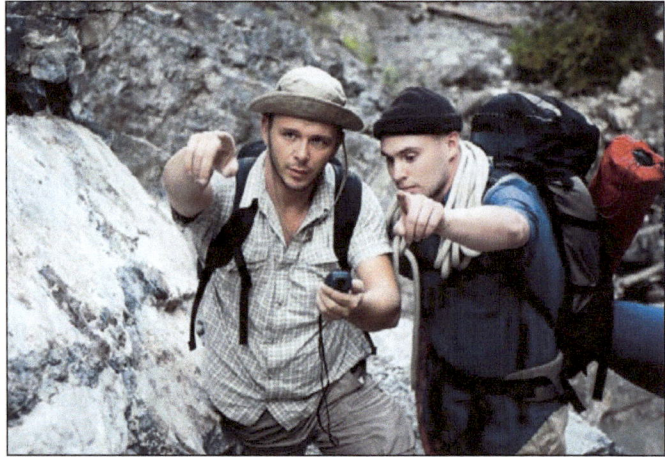

In chapters three to seven, I describe fundamental exercises that will foster improvement in power (Chapter 3); endurance (Chapter 4); core conditioning (Chapter 5); coordination, balance, and agility (Chapter 6); and flexibility and range of motion (Chapter 7). While each of these exercises has been explicitly categorized into a single chapter, realize that most benefit multiple fitness components, simultaneously. This is precisely why they are useful for developing an integrated, functional fitness. Throughout, pay strict attention to form, because proper execution is critical to your ability to do the exercises efficiently and safely.

This list of exercises is meant to be representative and is by no means exhaustive. As a trainer, I constantly watch, ask about, and try new exercises. I am always looking for new tools that I can use in my own workouts and with my clients. I don't want to imply any ownership of the exercises covered in this book; I am only endorsing them. For additional exercises, three outstanding references are seanburch.com, Crossfit.com, and mtnathlete.com. I am a proponent of their approaches and applaud their dedication to functional fitness. Also, visit www.spartanfitnessalaska.com for video clinics on select exercises.

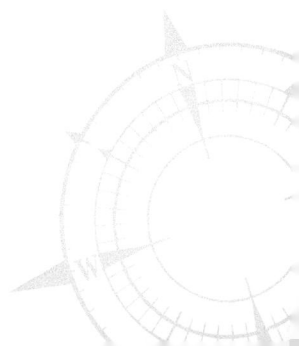

*"THE DIFFERENCE IS
ONLY ONE OF SCALE"*

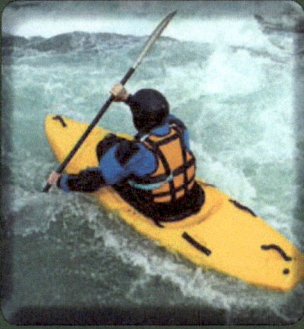

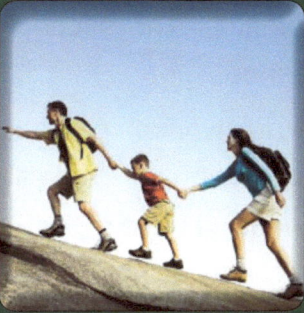

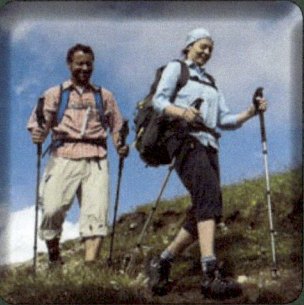

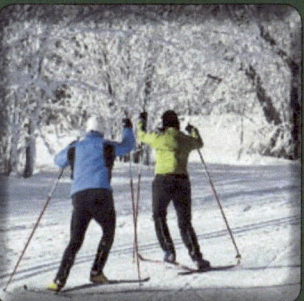

CHAPTER 2:
WHY FAILURE IS YOUR
FRIEND

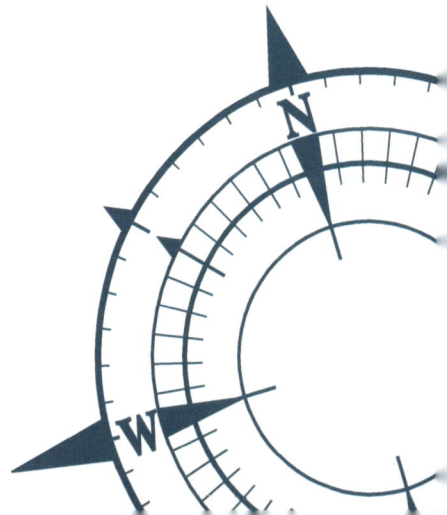

My son was born five weeks premature. He is generally in good health but one of the lingering effects has been some delayed motor development. We continue to see a physical therapist two times a week and focus on his hip flexor strength, balance, and knee and ankle posture.

The challenge he faces is twofold. The first challenge is physical. He needs to develop muscular strength, learn appropriate posture, and hone his kinesthetic awareness to achieve correct motor function when sitting, standing, walking, and running. The second challenge is more cerebral and relates to confidence.

My son's physical therapist is a wonderful woman named Joyce (imagine working as a physical therapist with two-year-olds all day …this alone should convey automatic sainthood). I have repeatedly learned tools and approaches I use with my clients by observing her interactions with my son. To help him develop the physical tools he needs, she must challenge him to try new things or to approach known tasks in novel ways. She pushes him to the edge of, and sometimes beyond, his comfort zone. As a parent, it can be difficult to watch, particularly when you see your child struggling or, even more heart wrenching, looking to you for help.

However, I recognize that he needs to be pushed. He can be pushed in a safe and supportive environment, but he needs to be pushed to counteract the effects of his delayed development now and into the future.

The lesson is that significant growth often arises from the most challenging of circumstances. This spans the physical, the emotional, and the spiritual. In the context of physical training, I want to encourage you to push yourself. Be willing to try new things. Be willing to fail. On multiple occasions, I have seen clients progress from doubtful looks, to reluctant willingness, to competency, to prideful tears. I have experienced this myself.

As you embark on the specifics of the training approach in the following chapters, I encourage you to adopt the following mindset: If human beings are capable of this task, and I am a human being, then I am capable of this task. You don't have to run as fast, jump as high, or lift as much as an Olympian. But you can run fast, jump high, and easily lift objects you encounter in daily life. The difference is only one of scale.

Many of the exercises in this guide are appropriate for beginning or deconditioned athletes. However the same exercises are appropriate for advanced individuals who have already achieved a high level of fitness. The appropriate scaling is achieved by increasing the range of motion, the weight moved, the speed at which the movement is performed, or the number of repetitions. Similarly, reducing the rest time between exercises will also increase intensity. Other movements are more advanced but can eventually be achieved by most anyone, particularly by developing proficiency in the smaller movements that make up the more complex skills. There is tremendous value in the practice of these advanced movements, even if little or no weight is used.

The advantage of building a foundation of fitness in a gym or other controlled setting is that it allows you to push your limits to increase your functional capacity in a safe environment. These benefits will translate to your recreational endeavors when you apply your broadened physical abilities to the trail, the slope, or the water, regardless of the activity or season, as you will be able to go faster, higher, and longer.

The most accomplished athletes in the world continue to train and practice their craft. They constantly push their own boundaries. They know they can always get better. This is true of us all.

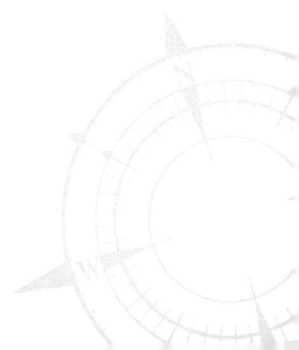

"WE WANT TO TRAIN FOR POWER, NOT JUST STRENGTH"

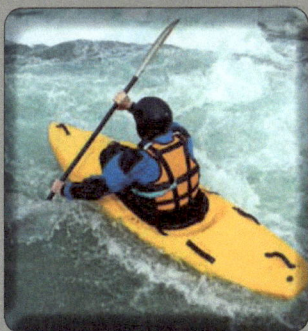

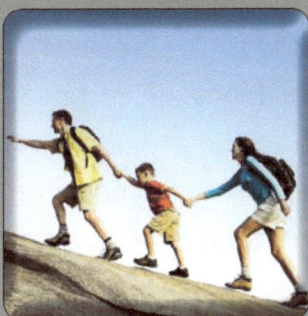

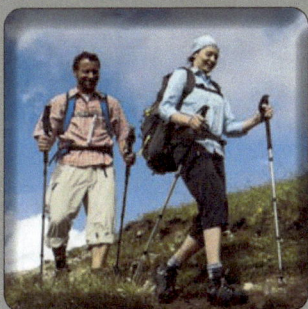

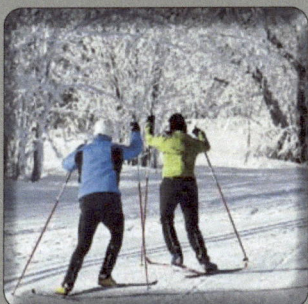

CHAPTER 3:
STRENGTH, SPEED, & POWER

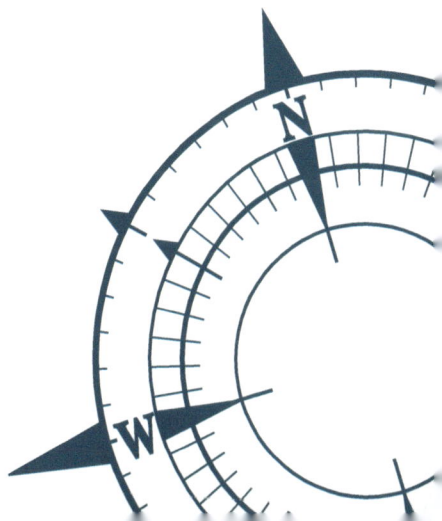

Practically speaking, strength is the ability to exert force, speed is the rate of motion, and power is the application of force over distance. In essence, power is the product of strength and speed. Functionally, power is largely what we use in everyday life. Power is how you drive up a slope when skate skiing, how you traverse a channel while kayaking, and how you lift yourself up onto a ledge when bouldering. We want to train for power, not just for strength.

To illustrate this point, let's consider two pieces of equpiment commonly used to develop strength in the upper legs: the leg extension machine and the hamstring curl machine. Many of us have logged hundreds, if not thousands of repetitions on these old standbys. For those of you unfamiliar with them, a leg extension machine is basically an elevated chair. Some form of resistance is located roughly at ankle height or just above. With your hips and knees fixed in space, you raise your feet until your legs are straight. This movement is achieved through the contraction of the muscles on the front of your thigh (quadriceps) and stimulates muscle growth and strength development.

A hamstring curl machine is basically a bench on which you lie face down with the resistance centered behind and slightly above the ankle joint. You curl your heel towards your glutes (backside), starting from a straight leg position and ending with a roughly 90° angle between your upper and lower leg. Again, the hip and knees are fixed in position and the muscles on the back of the thigh (hamstrings) are responsible for the movement and are stimulated relative to strength and size.

Leg extensions and hamstring curls are effective at increasing strength and muscle mass but are inefficient at developing functional power. This is because these two muscle groups are designed to work together, in unison with the muscles of the hips, lateral and medial leg muscles, core, and lower leg. It makes little sense to train them separately. To drive this point home, try to think of a single task in daily life or a common recreational activity that requires or employs a hamstring curl as performed in the gym. I am guessing this will leave you stumped.

Instead, we want to focus on developing power that translates outside the gym. To do so, we should try to replicate functional movement. This will train the body to move, generate inertia, and handle momentum as it was designed. Your body doesn't function as a collection of independent muscles and joints clumsily handing work from one body segment to the next like a bucket brigade fighting a fire. Instead, the body fluidly and efficiently transfers power generated in large muscles to smaller and smaller muscles. It is a highly orchestrated series of fulcrums and lever arms that can execute an endless variety of tasks in multiple planes. Further, training and using the body as designed is less likely to result in strains or other injuries; whereas imbalances can result from isolation training.

Rarely do practical movements span a single joint. In the examples above, the leg extension and hamstring curl require movement only at the knee while both the ankle and hip are fixed. Further, all of the movement takes place in a single plane (i.e., involves a forward and backward movement only, with no rotation). Almost any athletic movement requires movements across multiple joints and occurs in multiple planes.

As an example, envision a soccer player striking a ball. Strength is required to propel the ball forward. But, the speed and strength generated by the hips are what result in the tremendous power transferred to the foot and delivered to the ball. The ankle, knee, and hips of the lower body are all engaged and even the body's core and upper body play important roles in stabilization, balance, and momentum transfer. Finally, there is significant body rotation, thus the movement occurs in multiple planes.

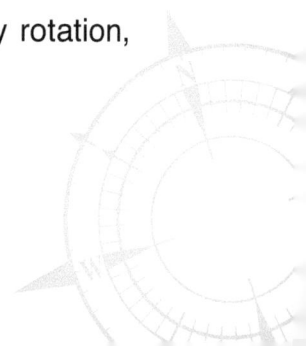

To develop functional power we largely want to select exercises that replicate, or at least enhance practical movements that span multiple joints. Further, we want to include some work that requires the generation and control of power in multiple planes.

Below I describe the fundamental power-training movements. For further detail and video demonstrations, visit www.spartanfitnessalaska.com to view clinics on specific exercises.

SQUATS

The squat is the single most fundamental functional movement of the human body. It is how you get up and how you get down. I recommend the squat as the foundation of any fitness program for any purpose at any age. You can squat heavy (e.g., 300+ lbs on a barbell on your back) or light (e.g., a medicine ball or just your body weight) and see endless benefits. It allows movement over multiple joints and is particularly effective at developing the functional ability to generate and transfer power from the hips.

Envision mountain biking upslope but in a low gear to maintain speed. The power you are able to generate and apply is greatly enhanced by squats. Similarly, stepping up over or onto rocks or bouldering, particularly when carrying a pack, requires significant leg and hip power and endurance. This is true on both the ascent, where you must lift your body against gravity, and the descent, where you must control your weight as you lower it to prevent injury. Because of the number of large muscles engaged and resulting increased oxygen demands, squats can provide cardiovascular benefits as well.

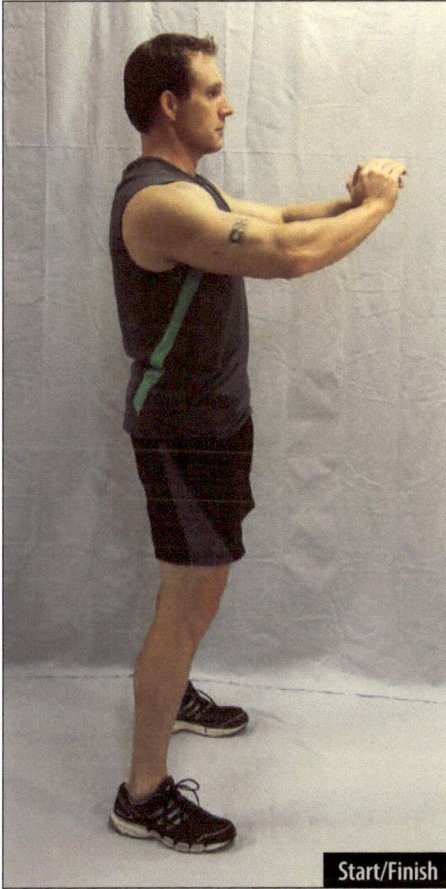

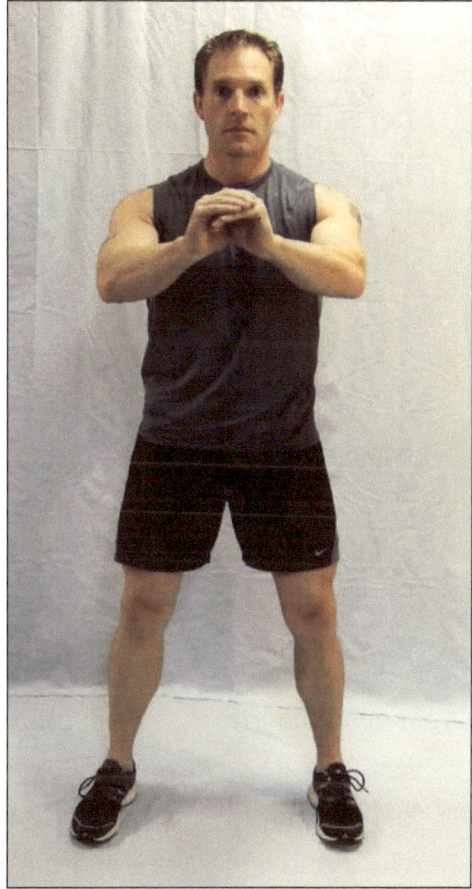

Start/Finish

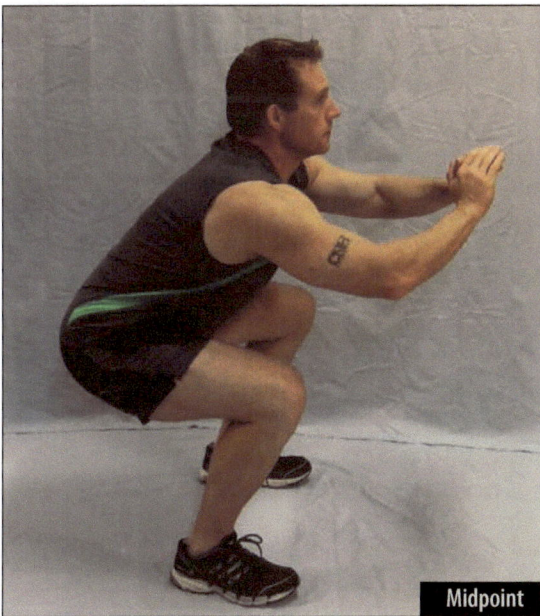

Midpoint

COACHING POINTS

1. Develop a stable base. Your feet should be just wider than shoulder width apart with your feet turned out 5° to 10°.

2. The distribution of weight across your foot should be centered directly over your lower leg (i.e., you should neither be on your toes nor on your heels).

3. Your head should remain level throughout the entire motion as this will protect your back by ensuring correct posture. If training with a mirror, focus your gaze on your reflection roughly at the level of your forehead. If no mirror is available, pick a point at eye level on the facing wall. Whether using your reflection or another guiding mark on the wall, maintain visual contact throughout the movement.

4. Your initial movement should be down and back with your hips, not forward and with your knees. To help envision the correct movement, imagine that someone has a rope tied around your waist and is pulling you from behind simultaneously backwards and down.

5. With heavy weight, your depth should be as low as you can go, while being able to comfortably return to a standing position. With light or no weight, go as deep as you are able and strive to increase your range of motion over time (see Chapter 7 for a more detailed discussion of squat depth).

6. Your upward movement is initiated by a powerful press against the floor. Envision trying to push the floor away from you. This initial press is smoothly, yet powerfully transferred to the hips. Here, envision slamming a door using your hips.

7. Throughout the movement, your core will remain contracted and your normal, upright back posture should be maintained.

8. Breathe in during the downward phase and out during the upward phase.

DEAD LIFTS

The dead lift is an often underappreciated and, unfortunately, underused exercise. People think dead lifts aren't for everyone as they tend to envision power lifters straining to lift bar-bending loads. In functional terms, a dead lift is the appropriate way to pick up any object from the ground, everything from a child to a bag of dog food to a cooler full of freshly caught fish. Similar to the squat, it has significant benefits for the development of hip and leg generated power, has significant cardiovascular benefit due to the large muscle groups engaged, and can be performed with heavy or light weights.

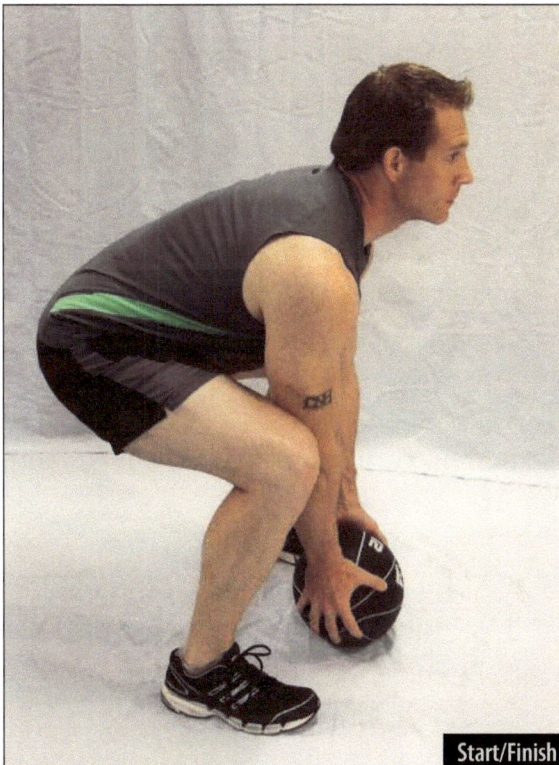

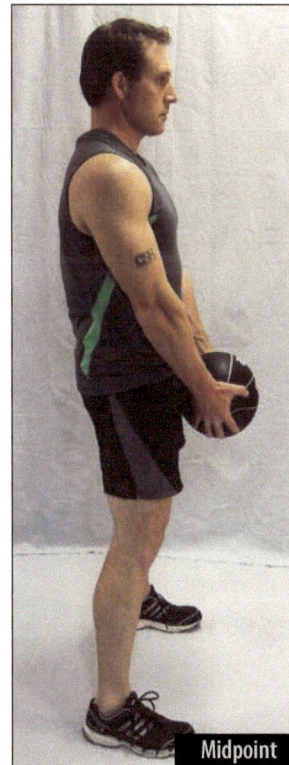

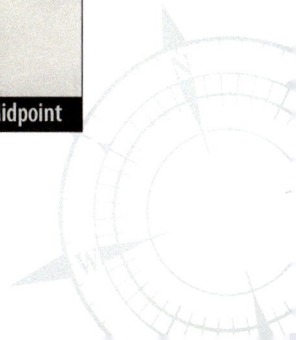

Start/Finish

Midpoint

COACHING POINTS

1. Develop a stable base. Your feet should be slightly narrower than a squat, roughly shoulder-width apart with your feet turned out 5° to 10°.

2. Your weight should be centered directly over your lower leg (i.e., you should neither be on your toes nor on your heels—you should be able to wiggle your toes throughout the duration of the movement).

3. Your head should remain upright with your gaze directed slightly below eye-level throughout the entire motion as this will protect your posture. Imagine a penny on the ground roughly fifteen feet in front of you and keep your eyes on this penny as you execute the lift. You don't want your head straining upwards or bending downward.

4. Your arms should be straight and vertical, in line with the weight, and perpendicular to the floor.

5. Your initial movement should be initiated with the legs, largely the butt (gluteus) and thigh muscles (quadriceps and hamstrings). Envision powerfully pushing the floor away from you.

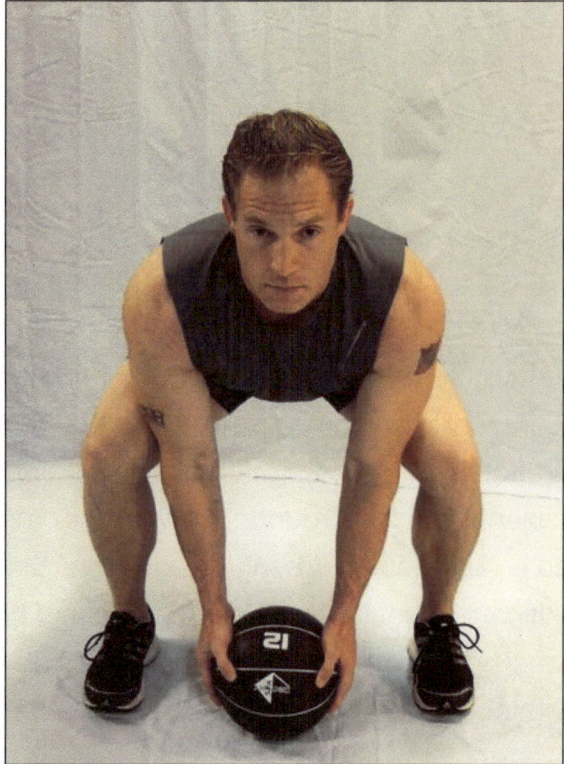

6. As you move the weight upward, the hips become engaged. Envision slamming a door with your hips.

7. As the power generated from the legs and hips drives the weight upward, the momentum will transfer to the back (latisimus) and shoulders (deltoids and trapezius) and you will roll the weight slightly back through your shoulders to a position of control.

8. The weight can then be lowered to the floor in the reverse order with the legs carrying the majority of the burden on the descent.

9. Be sure to maintain good posture on the descent as well as the lift.

10. The weight should be touching or nearly touching your body throughout the entire movement. Breathe in during the downward phase and out during the upward phase.

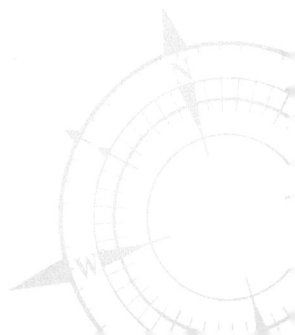

LUNGES

Lunges are an exaggerated stepping motion that challenges the upper thigh muscles of each leg independently. Lunges enhance lower body power, range of motion, and muscular endurance in activities such as trail running. Further, the lunge movement requires significant balance, relying on the muscles of the lower leg and the lateral and medial muscles of the hips and thighs. This is extremely useful in activities like skate skiing, which requires not only leg power but also balance to maintain the long, effective glide on alternating skis. Lunges can be performed using one's body weight, medicine balls, dumbbells, or barbells. In addition they can be performed in a forward stepping motion, stepping backwards, or at a slight angle to involve the inner and outer thigh muscles.

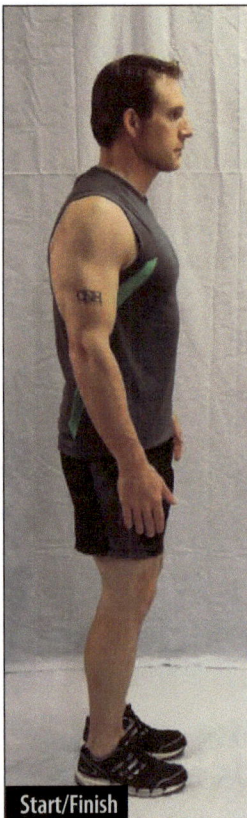
Start/Finish

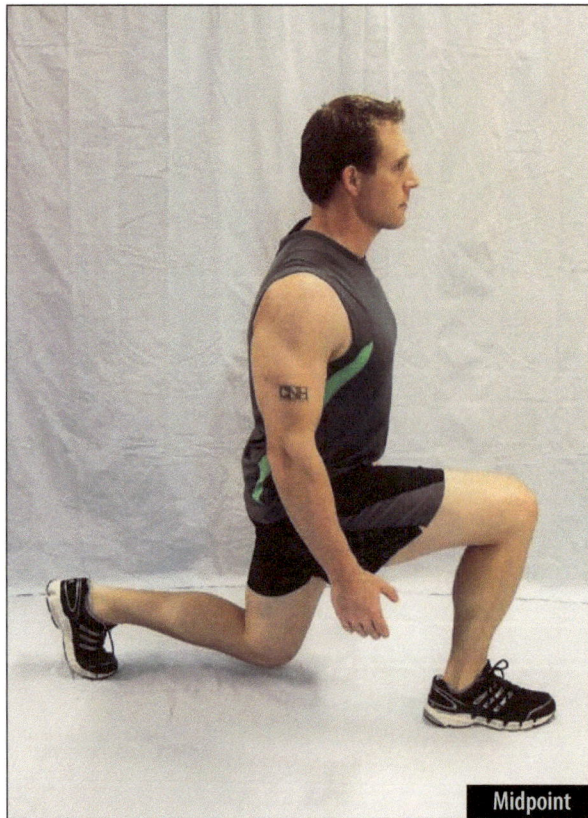
Midpoint

COACHING POINTS

1. Your stance should be similar to your normal standing position.

2. As you step forward, you want your stride to be slightly longer than normal, resulting in a 90° angle between the upper and lower leg of your forward leg, a 90° angle between the upper part of your forward leg and your torso, a 90° angle between your two upper legs, and a 90° angle between the upper and lower leg of your trailing leg.

3. Do not exaggerate the movement. Thus, do not hyperextend the trailing hip or allow the knee of the forward leg to move forward of the foot.

4. This movement involves both a forward step and then a controlled down and up motion.

5. The legs should be the primary muscles used to control your descent and drive the ascent.

CALF RAISES

Calf raises complement the power developed through squats, dead lifts, and lunges by utilizing the full range of motion at the ankle and strengthening the muscles of the lower leg. Calf raises will also enhance balance, especially at full extension of the foot. Calf raises can be performed on any step or platform.

COACHING POINTS

1. Stand such that your toes are securely placed on the surface but your mid-foot and heel movement are unimpeded.

2. Raise and lower your body in a slow and controlled manner through the full range of motion at the ankle.

3. Foot placement (toes pointed slightly inward, slightly outward, or straight ahead), external weights, and one leg raises can be used to provide variation and increased intensity.

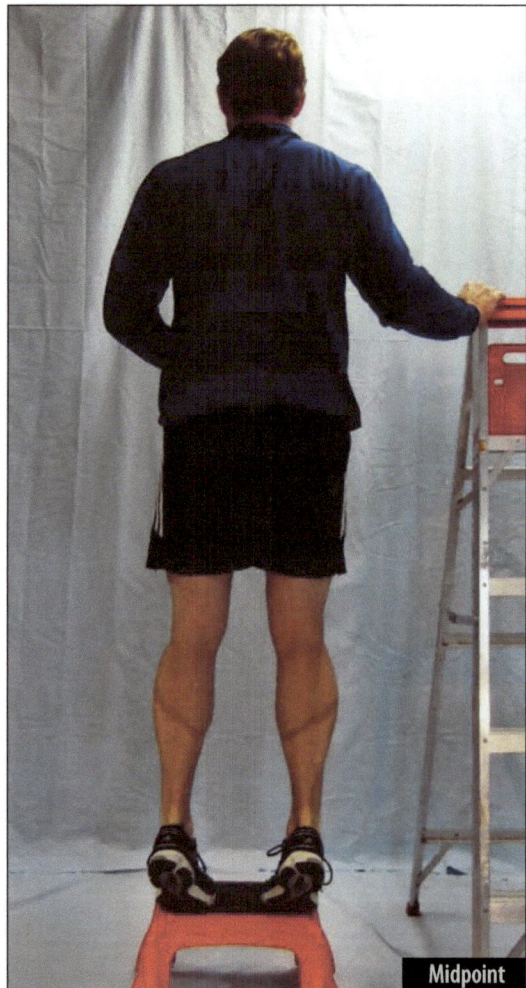

Midpoint

PULL-UPS/LAT PULL-DOWNS

Pull-ups are an outstanding exercise that engages all of the upper body muscles functionally used to pull (i.e., lift) your body mass against gravity. Any type of bouldering, rock or ice climbing, or swimming benefits greatly from enhanced upper body strength developed through a pulling motion. Specifically, the large muscles of the back (latisimus) are the major movers with assistance from the shoulders (rear deltoids, trapezius) and the front of the upper arms (biceps). Because many individuals can not complete a large number of repetitions using their body weight, assisted pull-ups and/or lat pull-downs can be used to train the same muscles through the same pattern, but with reduced resistance.

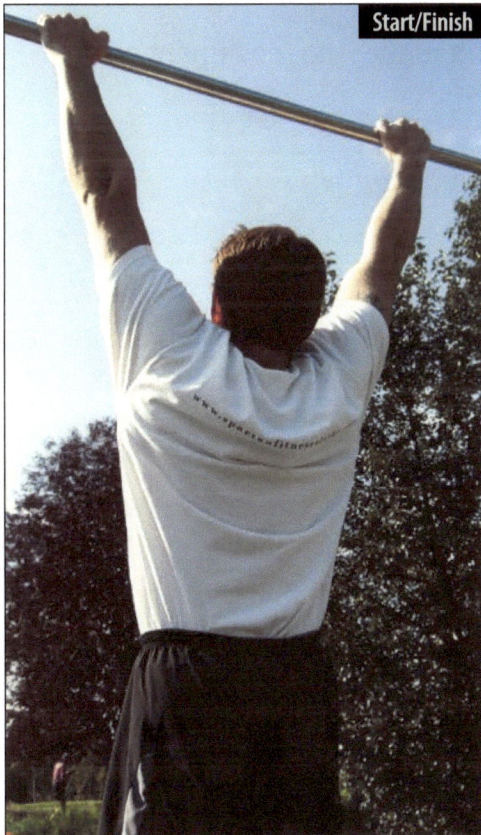

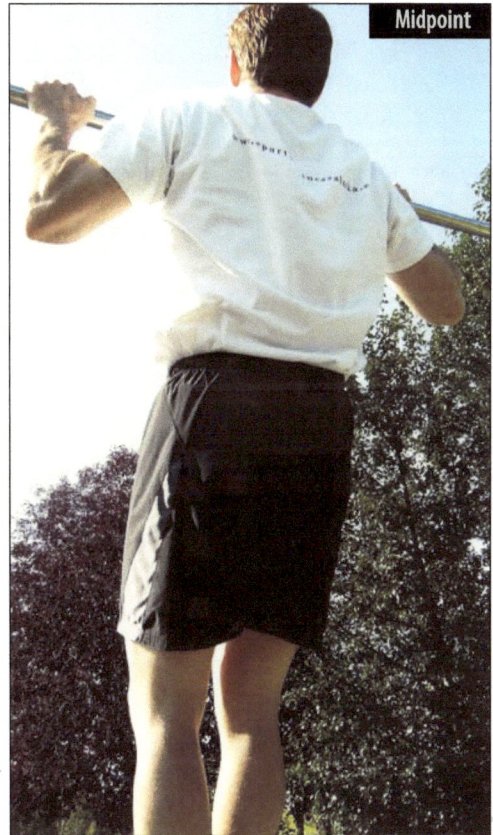

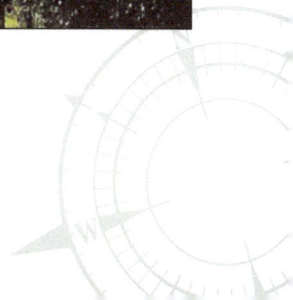

Start/Finish

Midpoint

COACHING POINTS (PULL-UPS/LAT PULL DOWNS)

1. Start from the downward position and allow yourself to relax your shoulder blades and hang, fully stretching your back and shoulders.

2. A variety of grips can and should be used over time.

3. Initiate the movement with the large muscles of the back. This momentum should then be smoothly transferred to and built upon first by the shoulders, then by the arms.

4. Continue the movement until your chin clears the bar.

5. After a momentary pause, lower yourself in a controlled manner to the full, stretched downward position.

6. Allow momentum to cease and repeat the movement.

ROWS

Rows train your body in the functional movement of pulling an object towards you (or your body towards an object if the object is heavier than you). Rows can be done in a variety of planes (perpendicular to gravity or against gravity), with a variety of tools (dumbbells, barbells, cable machines, etc.). Depending on the angle to the ground and the direction of pull, different muscles can be emphasized but the primary movers are the large muscles of the back (latisimus), the muscles of the shoulder (deltoids and trapezius) and front of the upper arm (biceps). This exercise certainly benefits any activities, such as kayaking or canoeing, that require this specific movement. In addition, strength developed in this plane will balance strength gained through pull-ups and through the pressing movements described below. Utilizing a variety of approaches is recommended.

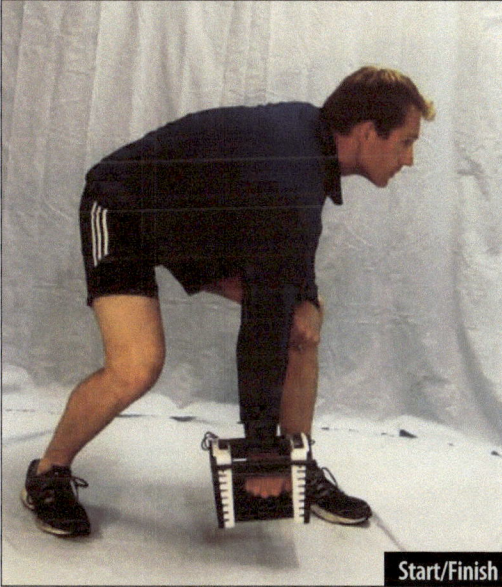

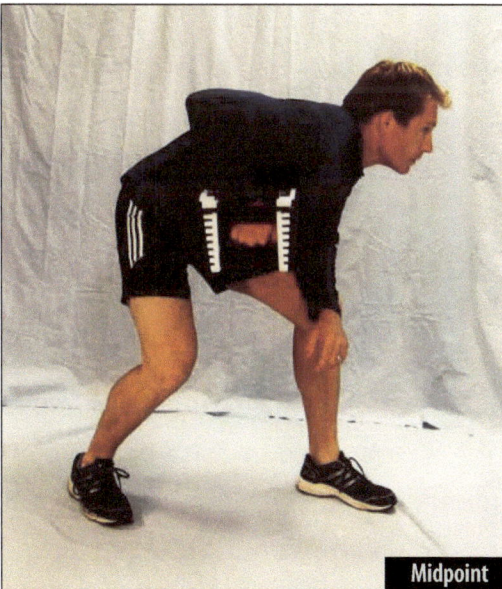

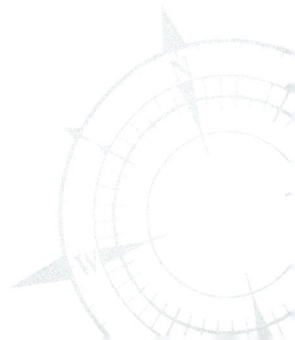

Start/Finish

Midpoint

COACHING POINTS (ROWS)

1. When performing standing upright rows, your stance should be similar to that of a squat with your feet slightly wider than shoulder width and your knees slightly bent to protect your lower back.

2. Ensure a full stretch of your back when extended.

3. Initiate the movement with the large muscles of the back (latisimus); thus the first movement should be in your shoulder blades, not your shoulders or arms.

4. Finish the movement by fully contracting the back. Envision trying to hold a pencil between your shoulder blades.

PUSHUPS/BENCH PRESS

The pushup and bench press functionally replicate the natural action of pushing an object away from you or pushing yourself away from an external object. In canoeing and kayaking, the use of a paddle or oar employs the coordinated combination of pushing and pulling movements. Power in the pushing motion is also important in the efficient use of poles when cross country or skate skiing. The primary muscles engaged are those of the chest (pectorals), shoulders (deltoids), and back of the arm (triceps); however, due to the balance required by both movements, additional muscles including the core and legs function as active stabilizers. Collectively, these muscles can generate significant functional power. The primary difference between the two movements is that pushups control one's body weight while the bench press requires control of an external object. Numerous variations exist for both movements including incline and decline bench press. Pushups can be modified by varying hand width, using grips to increase depth (i.e., range of motion), or resting on one's knees to reduce the resistance.

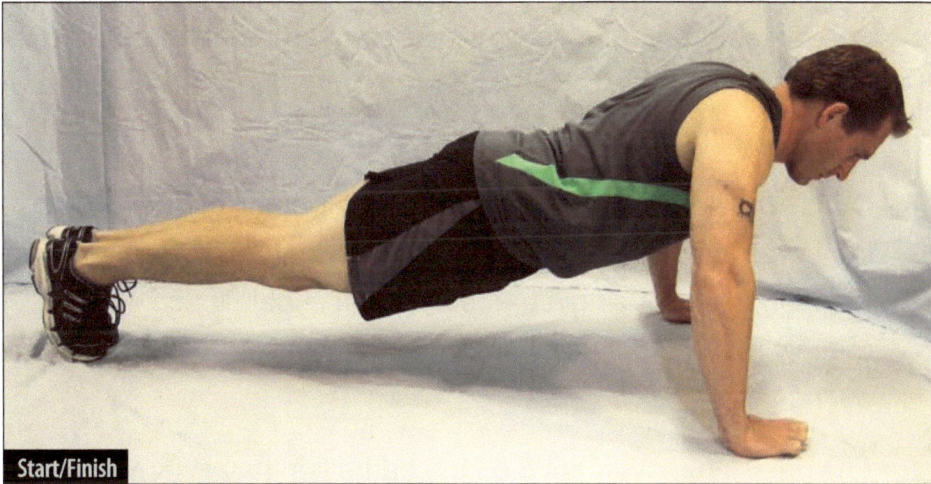

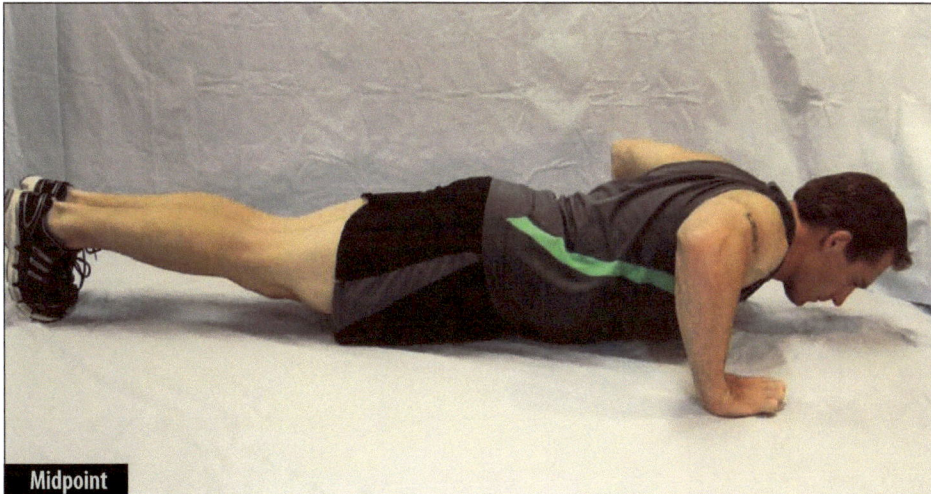

Start/Finish

Midpoint

COACHING POINTS (PUSHUPS/BENCH PRESS)

1. Focus on a stable base.

2. If doing pushups, your body should be a solid plank from the top of your head through your heels throughout the movement.

3. If doing presses lying on a bench, ensure your head, shoulders, and glutes are in contact with the bench throughout the movement. Similarly, keep your feet flat on the floor to balance your body.

4. During the negative movement (i.e., the barbell or the floor coming towards you), the angle of your elbow should break (be less than) 90°. When using a barbell, the bar should touch your chest roughly at a line drawn between your nipples. You should inhale during the negative phase.

5. The pressing movement (i.e., the barbell or floor is moving away from you) should be initiated by the muscles of the chest (the pectorals) rather than by your shoulders or arms.

6. When finishing the movement, straighten your arms to engage the back of the upper arm (triceps).

7. As a reminder, breathe out during the pressing movement.

SHOULDER PRESS

The shoulder press functionally allows one to lift an object overhead. The primary muscles utilized are the shoulders (deltoids) early in the movement and the back of the upper arm (triceps) late in the movement. Shoulder strength is important in a wide variety of activities ranging from climbing to rowing to skiing. In addition to enhancing performance, developing shoulder strength and range of motion has significant value in injury prevention as this joint is susceptible to painful and slow healing strains and sprains. Either barbells or dumbbells can be used to execute this functional movement and, ideally, it is performed in a standing position as this actively engages the core body muscles as stabilizers and more closely mimics practical movements.

COACHING POINTS

1. Use the same stance as for squats with a slight bend in the knees to protect the lower back.

2. Throughout the movement keep your wrist, elbow and shoulder in line vertically to ensure efficient lifting effort. Inhale during the downward phase.

3. When elevating the weight, fully press the weight upward such that your shoulder blades and shoulders are fully extended, as if reaching for the sky. Exhale when pressing the weight upward.

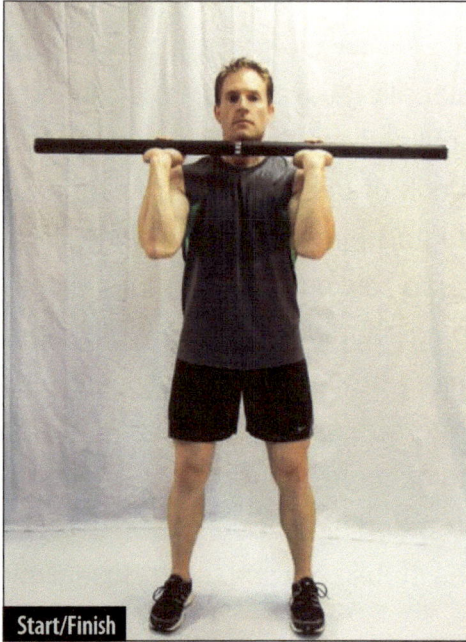

Start/Finish

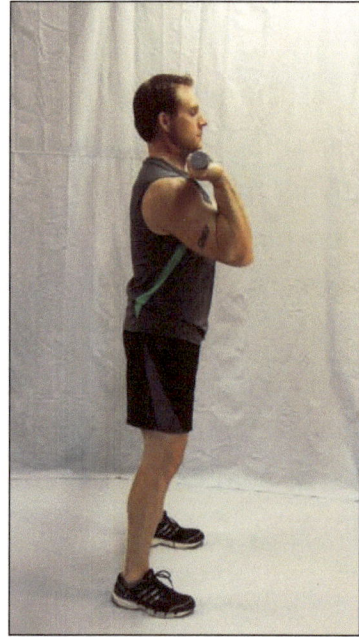

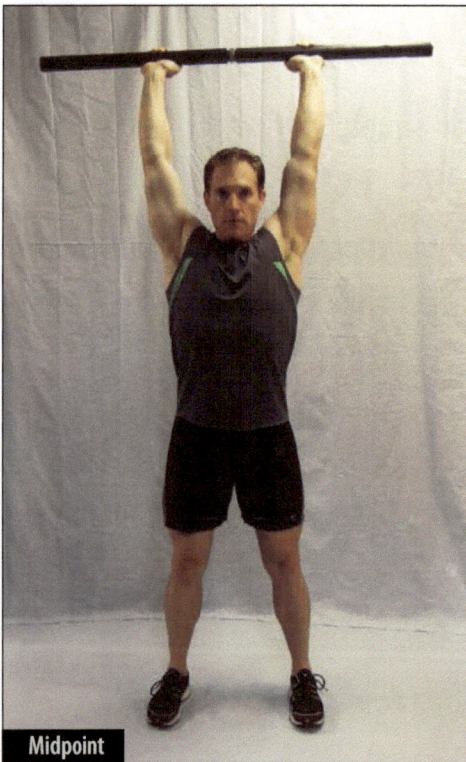

Midpoint

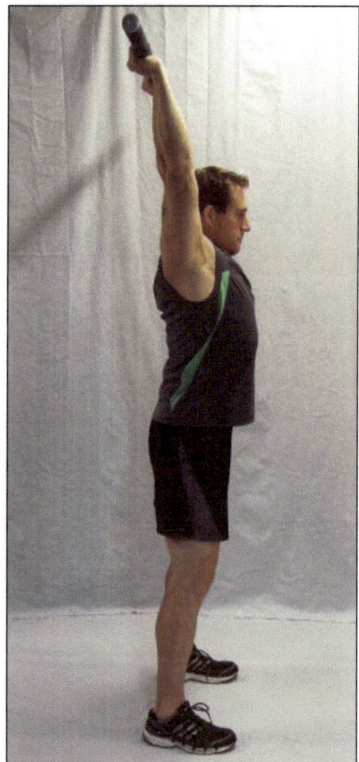

DIPS

Dips train you to lift your full-body weight against gravity using a pressing motion. This movement is very applicable to the powerful end phase of the poling motion used by both cross country and skate skiing and the end of several common swimming strokes. Similarly the end of a strong paddling motion heavily relies on shoulder and arm strength. Your chest (pectoral), shoulders (deltoids), and rear upper arm (triceps) are the active movers in this exercise. Typically, dips are performed using one's body weight but assisted dips allow for decreased resistance. Additional weight can be added using a hip belt for increased resistance.

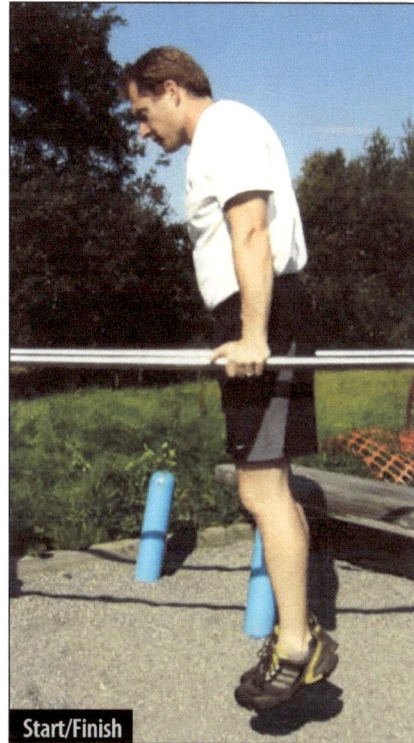

Start/Finish

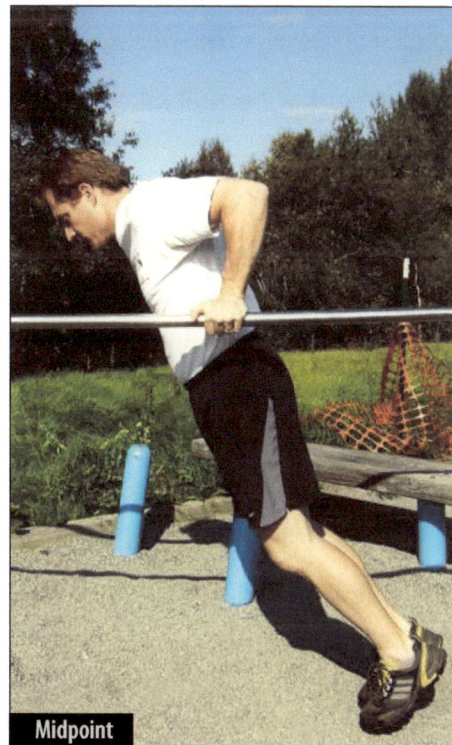

Midpoint

COACHING POINTS

1. When lowering your body weight, the angle of your elbow should break (be less than) 90°. The result is your shoulder being slightly lower than your elbow at the bottom of the movement.

Remember to inhale during this phase.

2. Exhale when pressing your body weight upward and completely extend your arms to fully engage your triceps.

FULL BODY POWER MOVEMENTS

The following three exercises combine multiple individual functional movements. The advantage of practicing these movements is their real world practicality (i.e., lifting an object from the floor to chest height and then overhead). For example, imagine lifting your kayak and putting it on your roof rack. Further, because they require the use of large muscle groups of both the upper and lower body, significant oxygen is required, resulting in aerobic and anaerobic benefit. The core muscles of the body are actively and functionally engaged as they serve not only to stabilize, but also transfer power from the lower body to the upper body. Finally, practicing complex movement is beneficial to overall coordination and body awareness.

POWER CLEANS

The functional use of the power clean is lifting a relatively heavy object from the ground to the chest position, such that your arms are underneath the object, allowing you to place the object or lift it overhead. It is, in essence, a dead lift coupled with a squat. My fifteen-year-old dog, Mickey, continues to accompany us on hikes, but his aging hips require that we lift him into and out of the back of our SUV. In essence, this is a 70 lb power clean. This is a very effective movement that is both practical and offers significant training benefit.

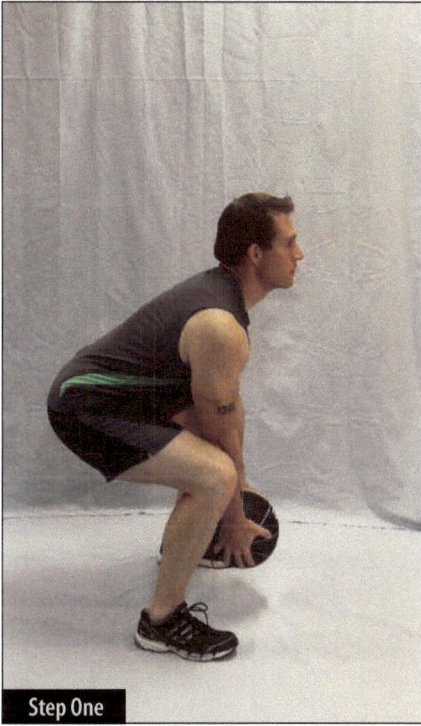

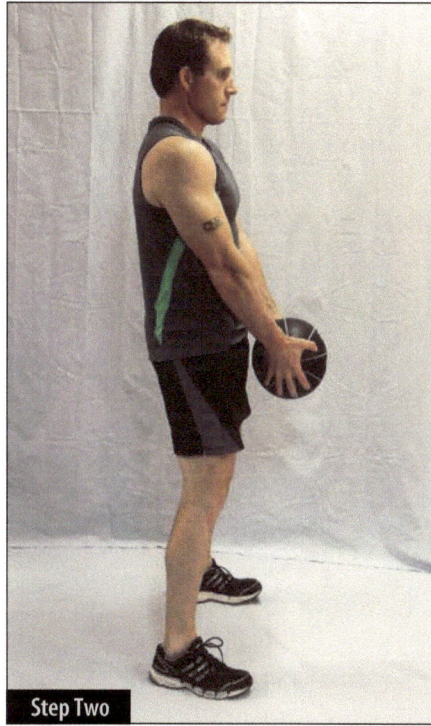

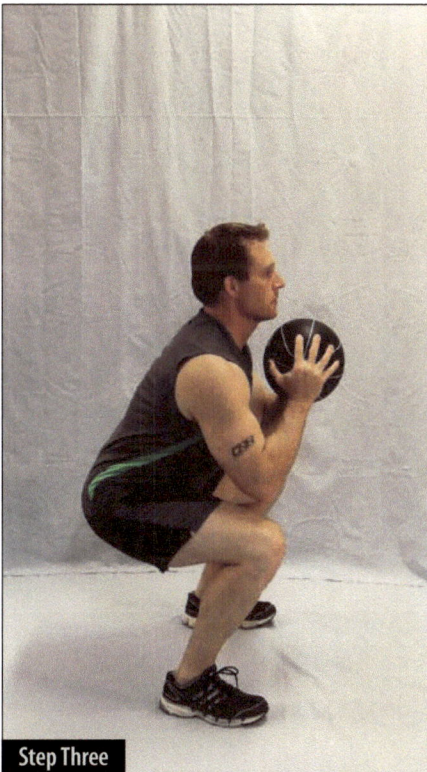

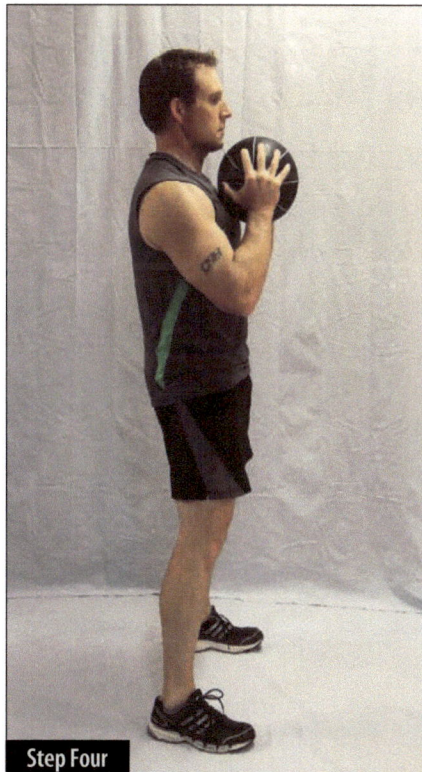

COACHING POINTS

1. Start in a dead lift position after reviewing the dead lift coaching points provided earlier in this chapter.

2. As the hips engage, driving the weight upward, initiate a shoulder shrug. However, rather than the shrug lifting the weight higher, use the shrug to pull yourself under the weight.

3. As you pull yourself under the weight, arrive in a squat position such that the weight is securely held by your hands with your arms underneath and in control of the weight. The weight should be located roughly at the height of your collarbone.

4. Execute a squat to finish the movement.

5. When the movement is complete, return to the beginning dead lift position.

6. During the entire movement, keep the weight close to your body. The path the object follows should be as vertical as possible.

7. Control your breathing throughout the movement due to the high oxygen demands.

THRUSTERS

A thruster is the combination of a squat with a shoulder press. The power initiated with the squat is carried through and added to by the shoulder press. It should be performed as one fluid movement rather than two distinct movements performed in sequence. A power clean combined with a thruster would be the appropriate way to move a heavy object from the ground to an overhead position (e.g., swapping a bin of winter gear for summer gear from the floor of your garage to an overhead shelf).

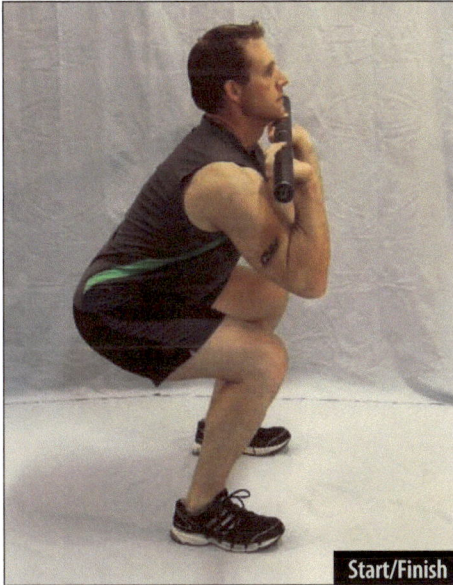

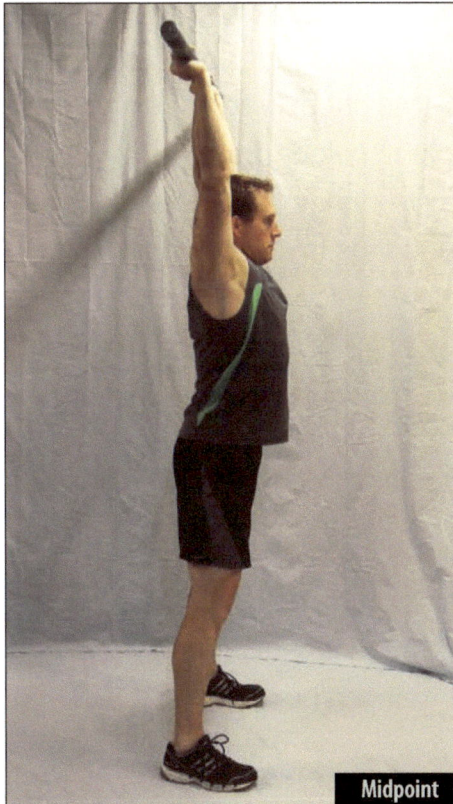

Start/Finish

Midpoint

COACHING POINTS:

1.   Start in a downward squat position with the weight located at collarbone height. Your arms should be below the bar with your hands securely holding the weight.

2.   Just as with a squat, the movement is initiated powerfully with the legs followed by the hips.

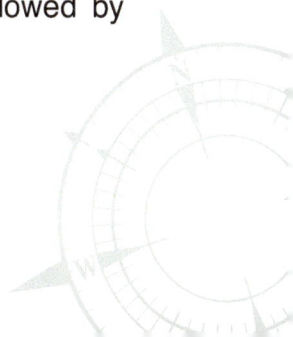

3. As the hips engage, the shoulder press is initiated resulting in a fully extended shoulder press.

4. When performed correctly, the weight is elevated upward so powerfully by the legs and the hips that it almost floats upward and is largely weightless against the shoulders and arm until much of the shoulder press movement is complete.

5. Similarly, if done properly, your feet will almost leave the ground.

6. The path of the weight should be nearly vertical.

7. Once in the upward position, reverse the movement, returning to the starting position with your legs receiving the weight.

PUSH PRESSES

Push presses are the result of engagement of the hip flexors, which generate and transfer power to a shoulder press. Most individuals can safely lift 2–3 times more weight overhead using a push press movement rather than a simple shoulder press. Functionally, this movement is the appropriate way to lift heavy objects from chest height to an overhead position. Canoe trips involving portages benefit from good form and functional power in the push press.

COACHING POINTS

1. This movement is identical to the shoulder press with one major exception.

2. The movement is initiated with a quick, explosive dip and drive of the hips that adds significant power to the movement and greatly increases the amount of weight that can be lifted overhead.

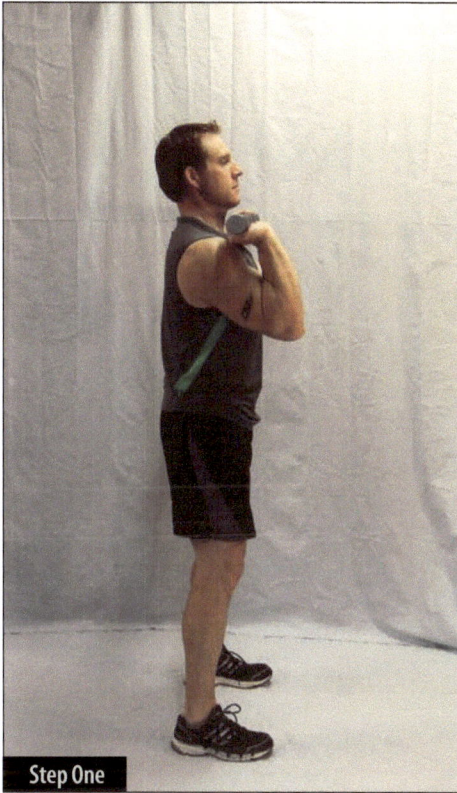

Step One

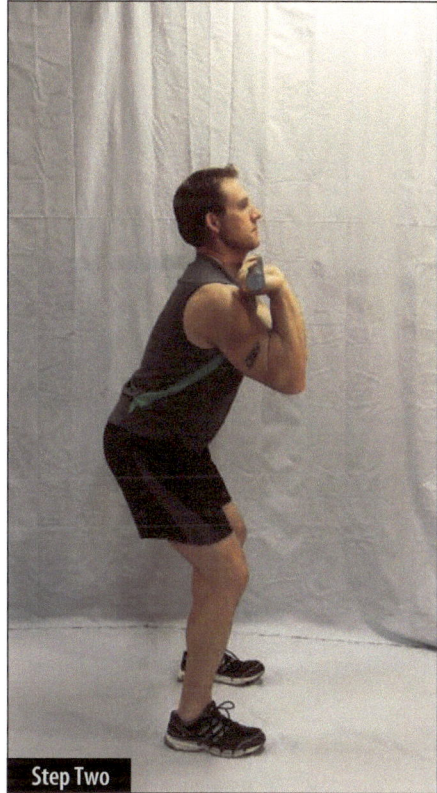

Step Two

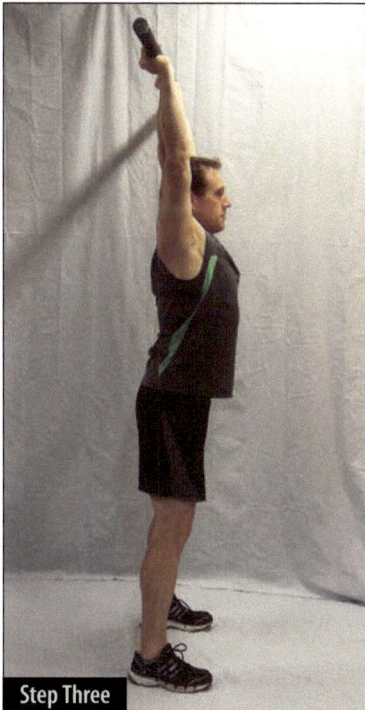

Step Three

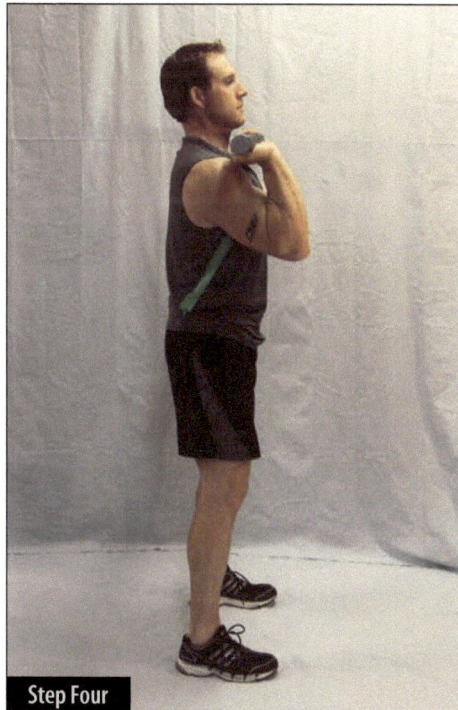

Step Four

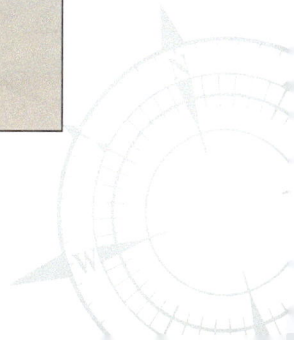

"THE EFFICIENCY OF ALL
THREE METABOLIC PATHWAYS...
CAN BE IMPROVED
THROUGH TRAINING"

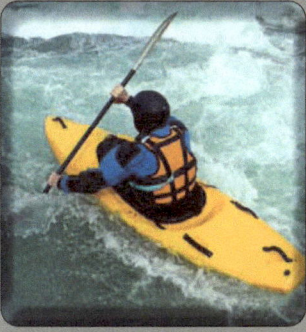

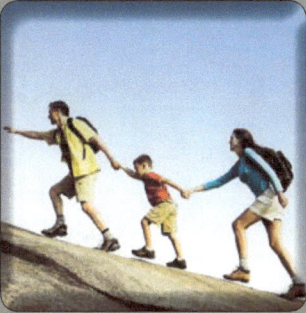

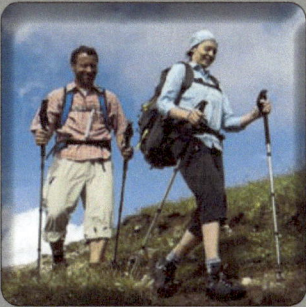

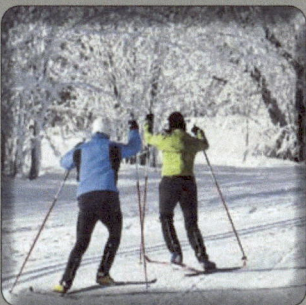

CHAPTER 4:
CARDIOVASCULAR & MUSCULAR ENDURANCE

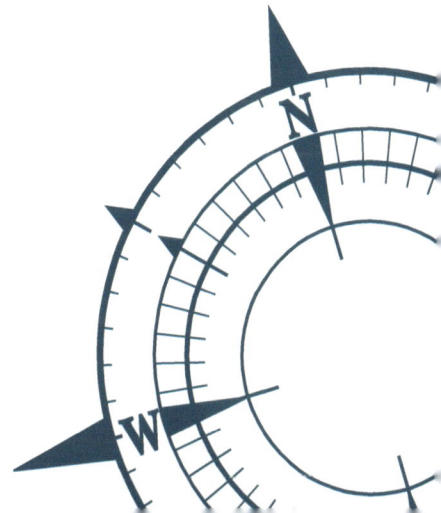

The term "cardio" usually refers to exercises designed to improve cardiac (i.e., heart) function. In essence, your body requires constant delivery of oxygen and nutrients to your working muscles as well as removal of metabolic byproducts. These transfers occur through the blood, which is delivered by the pumping action of the heart. These demands are increased during exercise and training benefits cardiac efficiency by increasing stroke volume (the amount of blood pumped per beat). Due to this increased efficiency, trained individuals have lower heart rates both at rest and during activity than untrained individuals. Despite the reduced heart rate, the increased stroke volume results in increased cardiac output (the amount of blood delivered per unit of time), thus improving the efficiency of nutrient delivery and waste removal and, ultimately, your ability to perform.

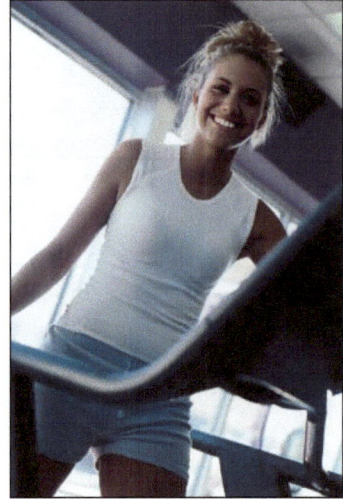

Another way to look at endurance is in the broader context of the three metabolic pathways that supply energy for muscle contraction, since this is the ultimate function we are looking to improve through training. The aerobic energy system requires oxygen and utilizes glucose, fatty acids, and amino acids. The glycogen–lactic acid system does not require oxygen (i.e., is anaerobic) and utilizes glycogen stored in the muscles. Finally, the phosphagen energy system uses adenosine triphospate (ATP) and phosphocreatine and is also anaerobic.

From a functional standpoint, long duration, low intensity activities rely almost exclusively on the aerobic energy system. Very short duration (e.g., 10–15 seconds), high intensity (e.g., maximum squats) bouts of activity engage the phosphagen system. The glycogen–lactic acid system is utilized for activities that are intermediate in duration (30–40 seconds) and intensity. The glycogen–lactic acid system and the phosphagen system can provide energy very quickly, but the stores utilized are also limited and quickly depleted. The aerobic energy system requires some time to engage but the energy stores are more plentiful. Thus, lower intensity activities can be maintained longer. Additionally, only 20% of the energy released aerobically goes to support muscle contraction while the remaining 80% is released as heat.

The point critical to us is that the efficiency of all three pathways and, therefore, one's performance when tasking each pathway, can be improved through training. Thus, we can and should include a wide variety of activities in our training. Further, we should vary the intensity and duration at which these activities are performed as an explicit part of our fitness program so that we address each of the three pathways. Mix in long slow sessions, shorter duration–higher intensity sessions, and interval sessions (single bouts with both high and low intensity; e.g., walk a block, jog a block, run a block, and repeat). This allows simultaneous training of both aerobic and anaerobic energy pathways.

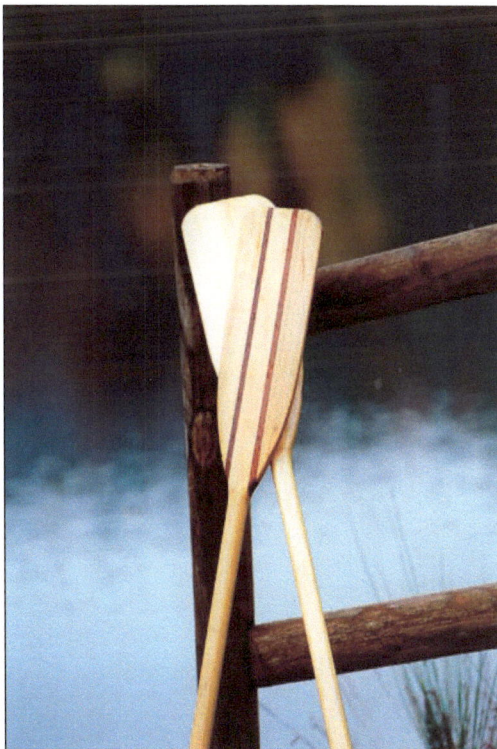

There are endless possibilities relative to cardiovascular and muscular endurance training. Traditional exercises or approaches such as running/jogging, biking, swimming, rowing, etc., all have the potential to significantly improve cardio-respiratory function. We

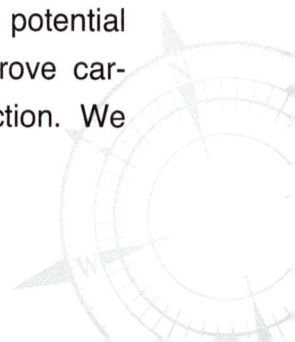

should especially include exercises that utilize multiple pathways simultaneously (e.g., skate skiing, hiking, or biking on variable terrain).

While all of these movements are, without question, functional, my recommendation is that one train in a variety of activities and mix in outdoor sessions as well. This will prevent the mental boredom that can come from over-structured or routine sessions. Developing competency in activities like climbing, skiing, ice climbing, and snowshoeing will broaden the tools available to you and allow you to span the seasons, regardless of the climate you live in. Workout diversity reduces the likelihood of injuries resulting from repetitive movements and fosters the flexibility benefits that come from engaging in a wide variety of activities through their full range of motion.

One common limitation most of us face is time. A functional and effective way to improve cardio-respiratory function is by performing the power exercises in the previous chapter and the agility and balance exercises in Chapter 6 at high intensity. Intensity can be increased by reducing the rest time between sets, increasing the rate

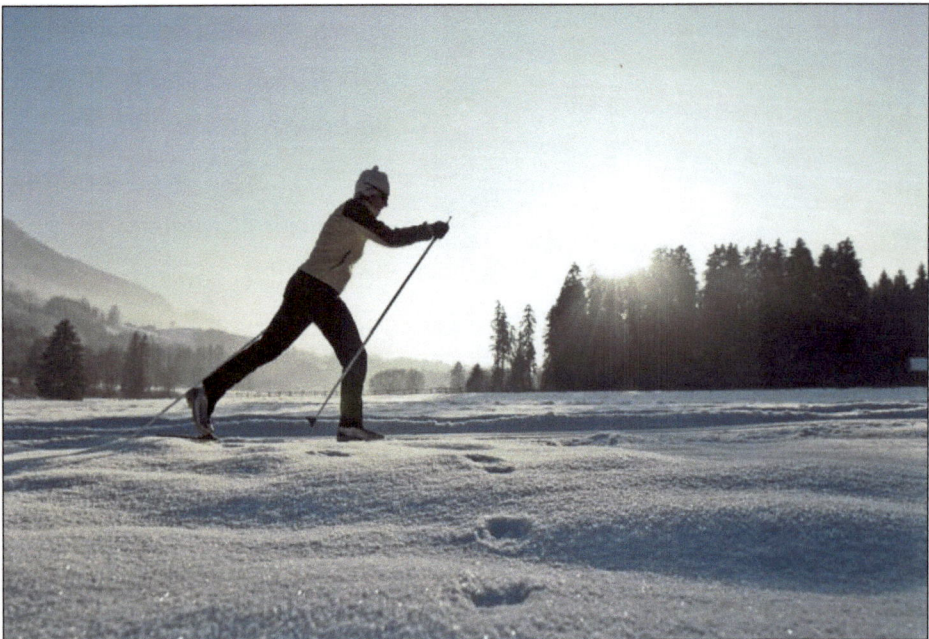

at which the exercise is performed (without compromising form), or increasing the resistance.

Whole body movements (e.g., power cleans, thrusters, power presses) are particularly effective in this regard due to the high oxygen demands of simultaneously engaging multiple large muscle groups. This approach to these exercises is, in essence, our holy grail as we are simultaneously training for power (Chapter 3) and aerobic and anaerobic fitness (Chapter 4). In addition, our core muscles (Chapter 5) are engaged as stabilizers and our balance (Chapter 6) is improved through the demands of controlling an external weight through a full range of motion (Chapter 7). Finally, due to the complexity of the movements, the communication and connection between the mind and body and one's kinesthetic awareness are improved.

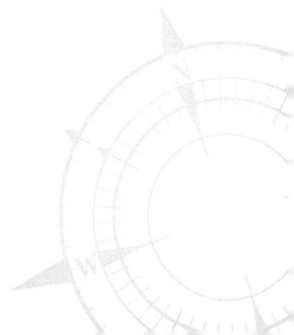

"CORE STRENTH IS CRITICAL
TO WHOLE-BODY FUNCTIONAL
PERFORMANCE"

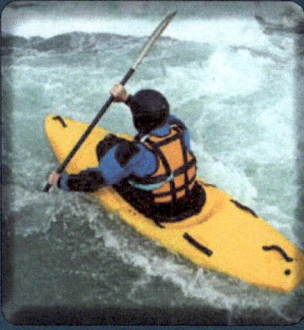

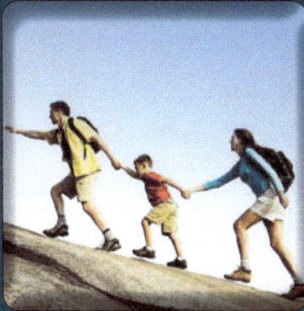

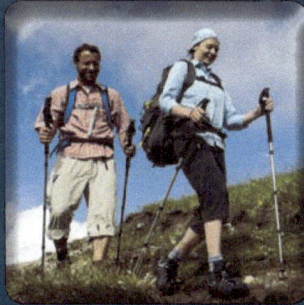

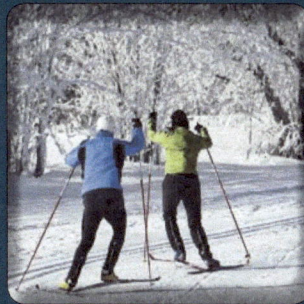

CHAPTER 5:
CORE CONDITIONING

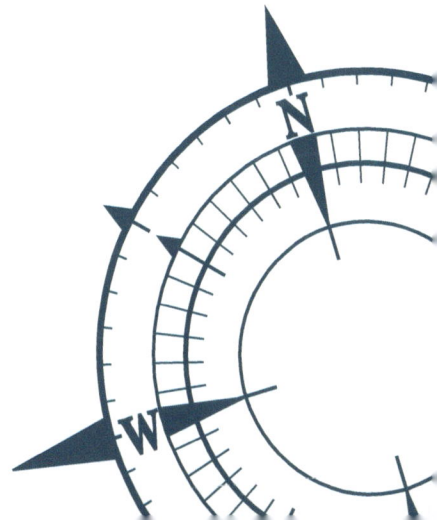

Core strength is critical to the functional performance of any dynamic activity. The core (including the hip flexors, lower back, and abdominals) stabilizes the body throughout any functional movement. This group of muscles is particularly important in movements that involve significant hip rotation (e.g., downhill skiing, some swimming strokes) or where a portion of the body is largely stationary (e.g., rowing and paddling).

The core also facilitates the safe and efficient transfer of power between the lower and upper body. When conditioned and used properly, the core not only maintains the momentum generated in one part of the body as it transfers this momentum to another part of the body, but adds to it. This is crucial to activities that require coordinated, whole body movements to efficiently drive propulsion (e.g., skate skiing, ice skating, rollerblading). Peak performance requires that the body function not as a series of largely independent muscle groups, but rather as one fluid and efficient organism. One instrument can't harmonize. Trained properly, your body can be a symphony. Core strength is critical to whole-body functional proficiency.

Many of the activities outlined in previous chapters and the chapters to follow engage and strengthen the core. These movements require the use of the core as a stabilizer and enhance their role in transferring momentum. Further, several of the exercises (e.g., squats, push presses) specifically develop the hip flexors' ability to generate power. Below, I have included several exercises that specifically train and increase the capacity of the hip flexors, lower back, and abdominals. Please visit the core conditioning video clinic at www.spartanfitnessalaska.com for demonstrations of these exercises.

ANCHORED ADOMINAL RAISES —

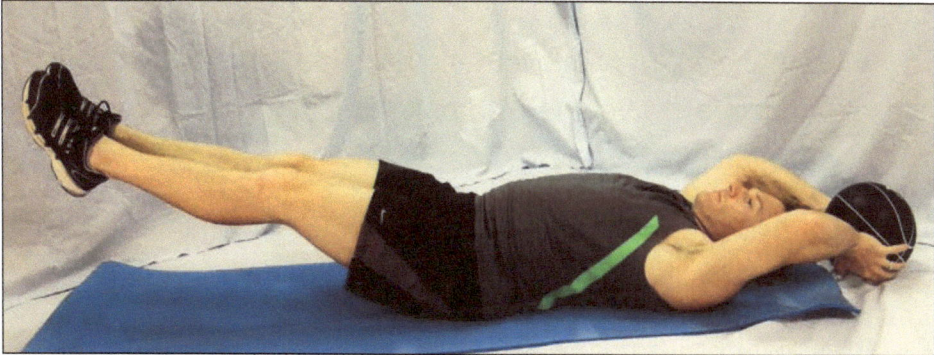

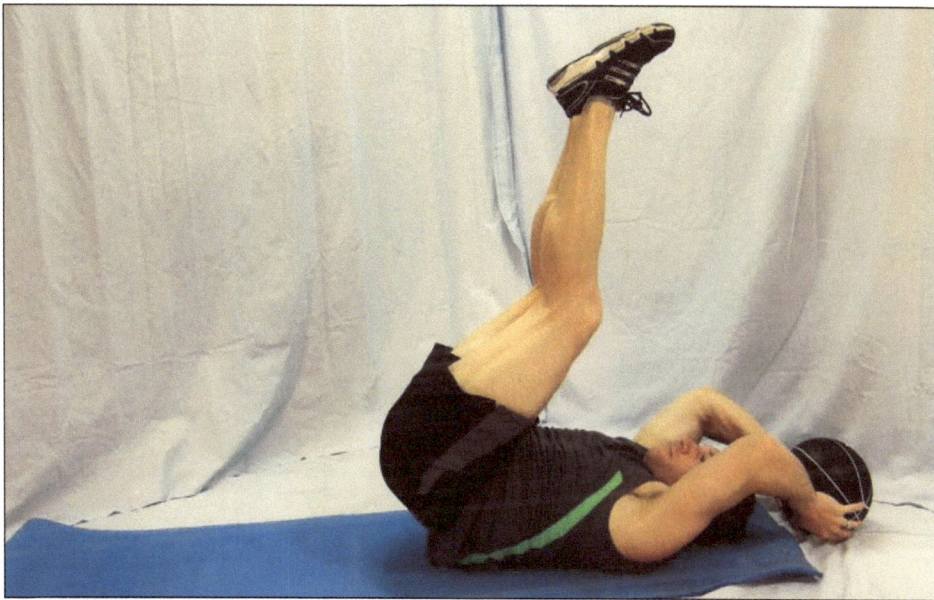

COACHING POINTS

1. Lie on your back and reach overhead gripping an object heavy enough to allow you to smoothly conduct this exercise.

2. Keeping your legs largely straight, raise your legs such that your feet are directly over head using your abdominal muscles and your hip flexors.

3. Slowly lower your legs again until your feet are a few inches off the ground and repeat the movement.

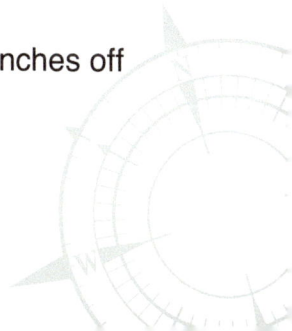

WWW.SPARTANFITNESSALASKA.COM

ABDOMINAL RAISES — COACHING POINTS

1. While hanging from an overhead bar or resting in an abdominal raise chair, allow your legs to hang freely with your toes generally pointed towards the floor.

2. Initiate an upward movement with your abdominals and hip flexors.

3. Bring your knees up towards your chest, pausing for and instant.

4. Slowly lower your legs to your starting position and repeat.

5. You can emphasize either your abdominals by slowing the movement down or your hip flexors by conducting the upward movement in a more explosive manner.

6. You can emphasize your obliques by slightly turning your hips to the side during the entire movement.

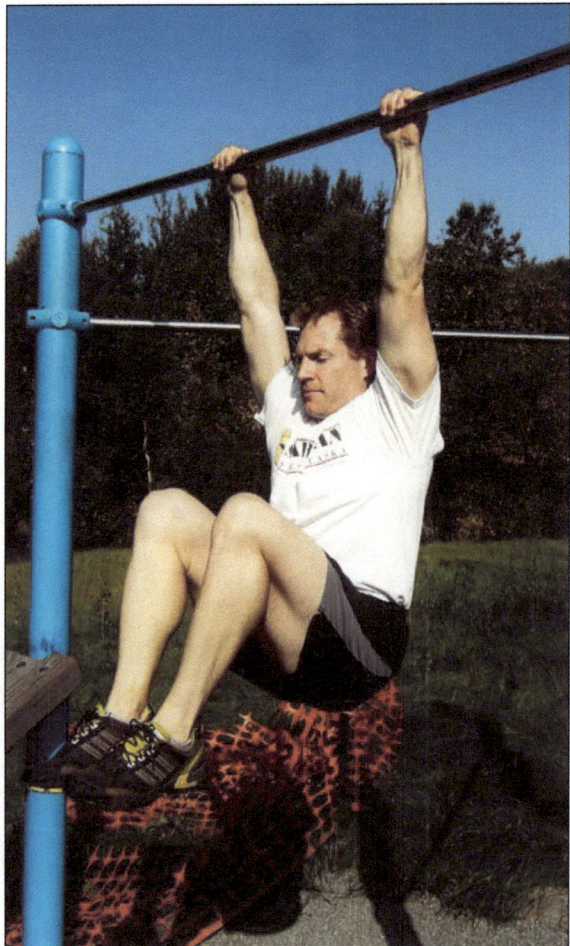

BICYCLES — COACHING POINTS

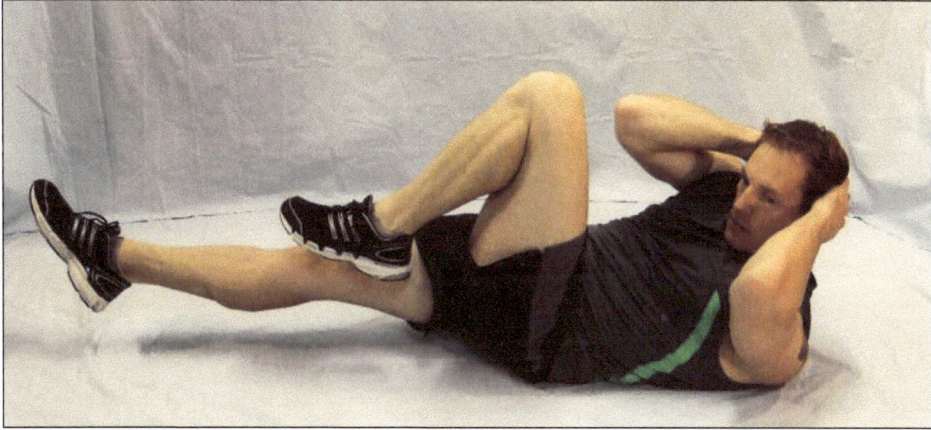

1. Lie on your back and bring your opposite knee and elbow together.

2. Lower both your leg and elbow and then repeat the movement with the other knee and elbow.

3. Throughout the movement, keep both feet and both shoulder blades off the ground.

4. Fully extend and point the toe of the strait leg as the other knee meets the opposite elbow.

5. The head should be resting in your hands. Don't "lift" your head using your hands. The abdominal muscles should do the work.

6. Conduct the entire movement in a slow and controlled manner.

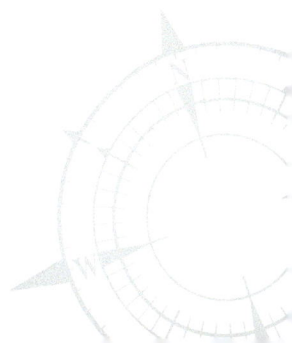

MOTH TO COCOONS — COACHING POINTS

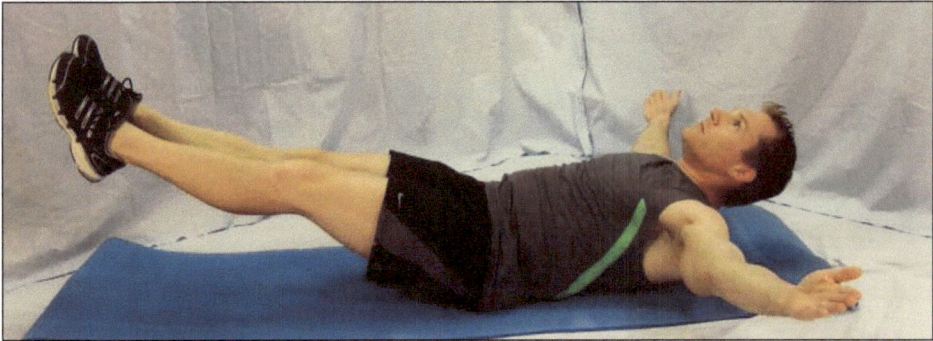

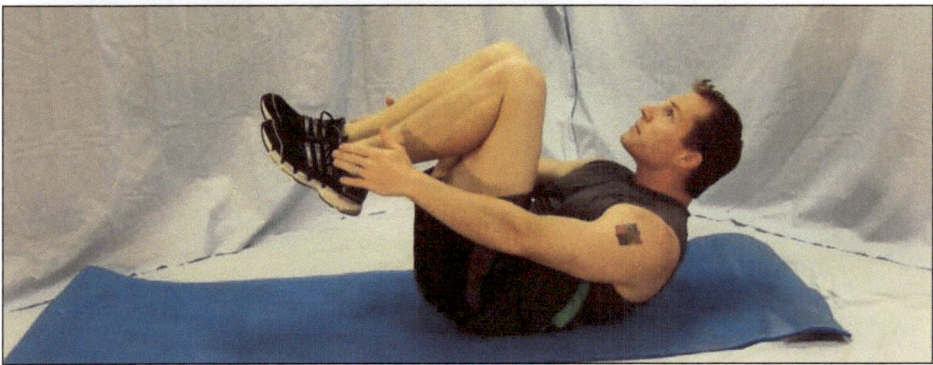

1. Lie on your back and fully extend your legs with pointed toes. Your arms should be fully extended to your sides. Envision being as large as you can.

2. Simultaneously bring your arms and legs together such that your hands end up next to your ankles. Envision being as small as you can.

3. Throughout the whole movement, keep your feet and shoulders largely off the ground.

4. Conduct the entire movement in a slow and controlled manner.

BIRD DOGS — COACHING POINTS

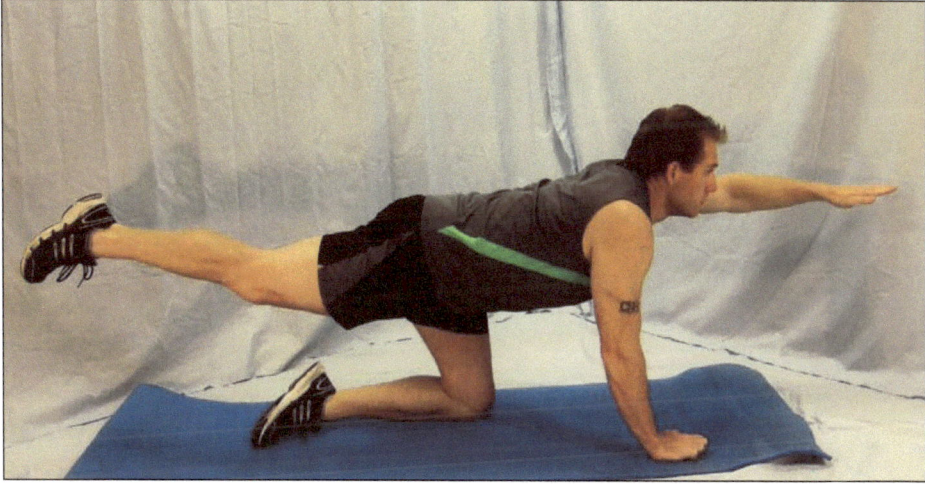

1. Position yourself on your hands and knees.

2. Raise your opposite arm and opposite leg fully extending both. You want to be as long and straight as you can from the tips of your fingers to the tips of your toes.

3. Hold this position.

4. Return to the starting position and repeat the movement using the other arm and leg.

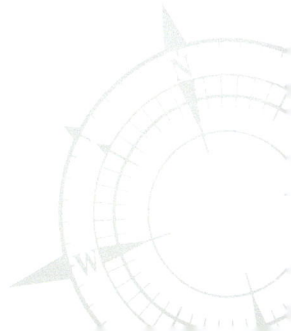

LYING BACK EXTENSIONS — COACHING POINTS

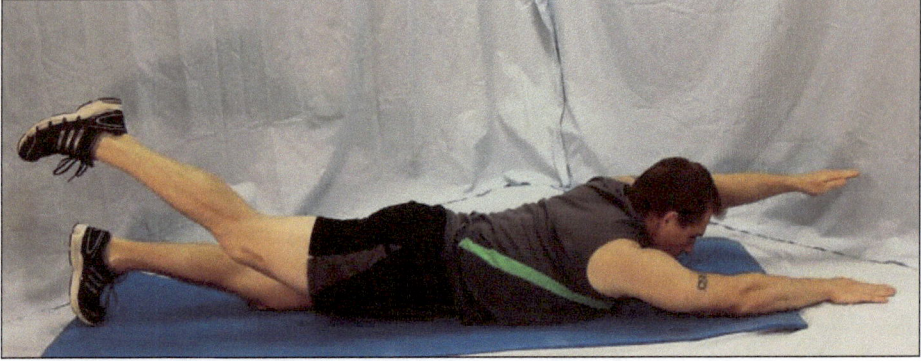

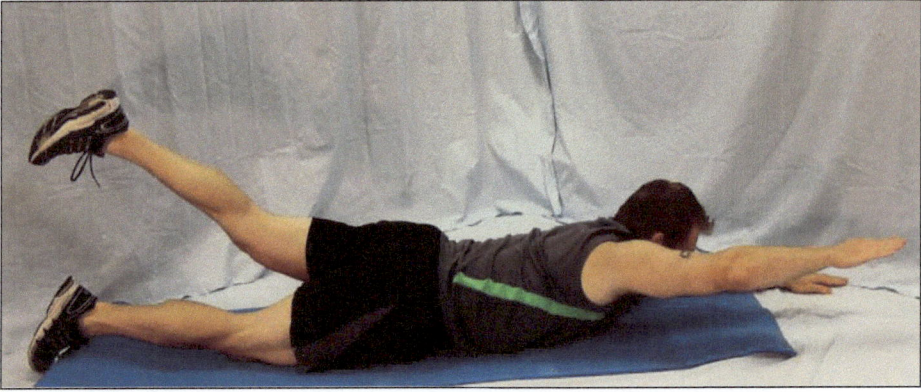

1. Lie on your stomach and fully extend both arms and both legs.

2. Raise your opposite arm and opposite leg 4-6 inches of the ground.

3. Hold this position.

4. Return the starting position and repeat with the other arm and leg.

STRAIGHT LEG DEAD LIFTS —

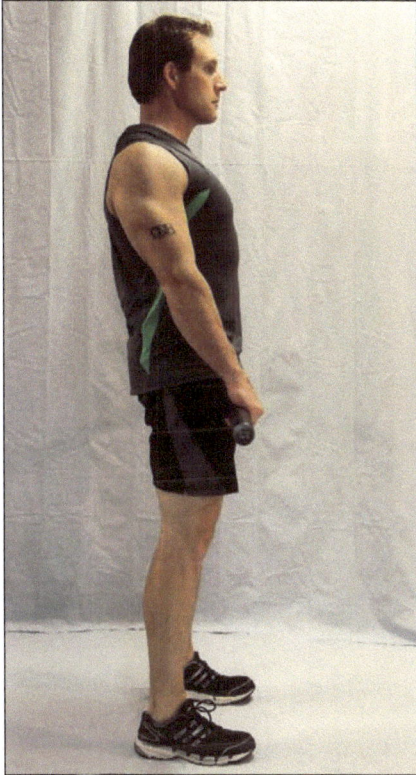

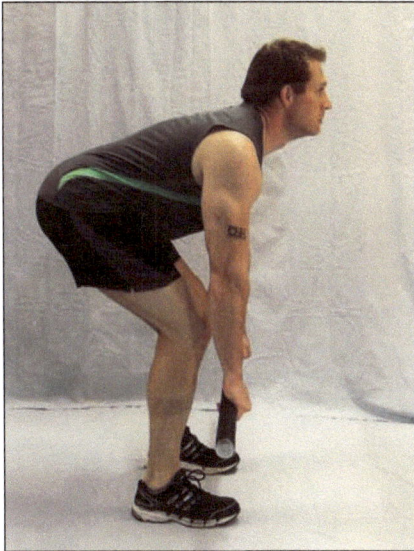

COACHING POINTS

1. Start in a standing position with a slight bend in your knees and holding a bar or object with straight arms. Start with a relatively light weight.

2. Initiate a slight backward movement with the hips and hinge at the waist.

3. Keep your head up, looking forward throughout the entire movement to maintain a straight back posture.

4. Lower yourself until your shoulders are level with or slightly below your waist.

5. Maintaining a rigid back, return to the starting position fully opening your hips.

6. Repeat the movement.

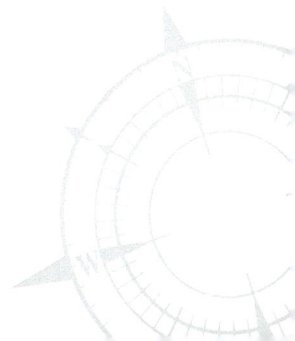

PLANKS — COACHING POINTS

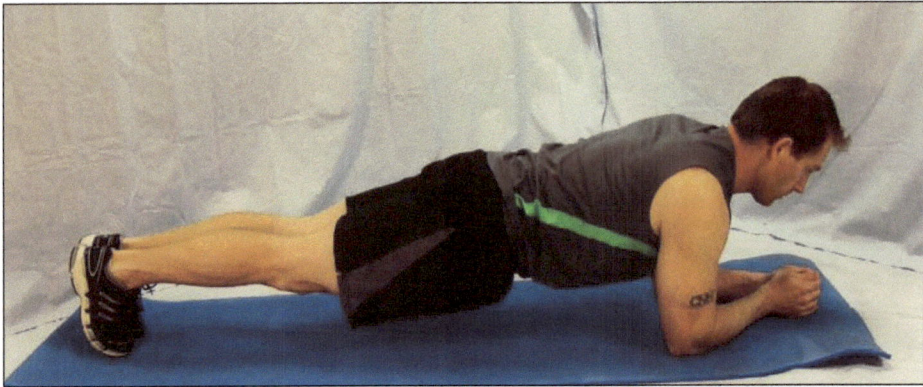

1. Face the floor and rest on your hands with locked arms or on your forearms.

2. Raise your hips off the floor and maintain rigid posture such that your body is straight from your shoulders to your feet. Your hips should be in line with your body.

3. Hold the position.

4. For increased intensity, raise one leg at a time and hold it.

SIDE PLANKS — COACHING POINTS

1. Face the wall and rest on your forearm or your hand.

2. As with a front plank, raise your hips off the floor and maintain rigid posture such that your body is straight from your shoulders to your feet. Your hips should be in line with your body.

3. Hold the position.

4. For increased intensity, raise your leg and/or your arm.

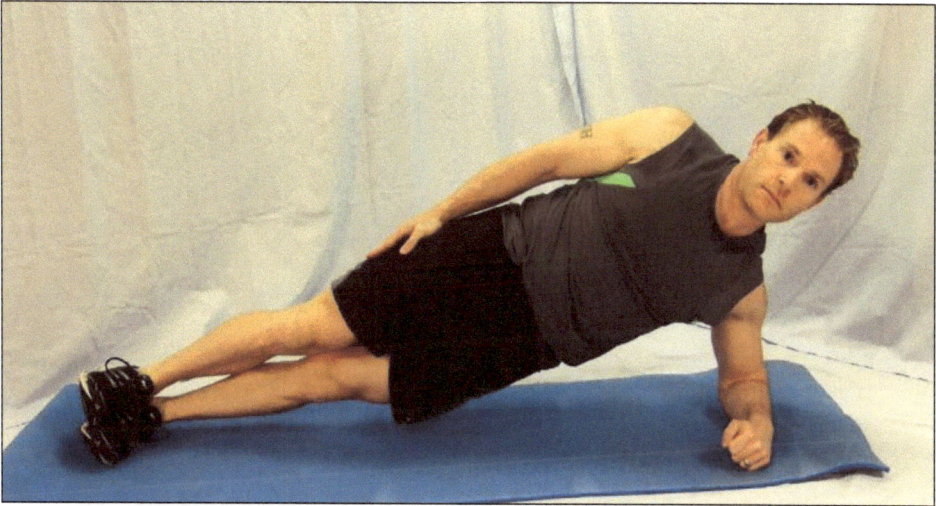

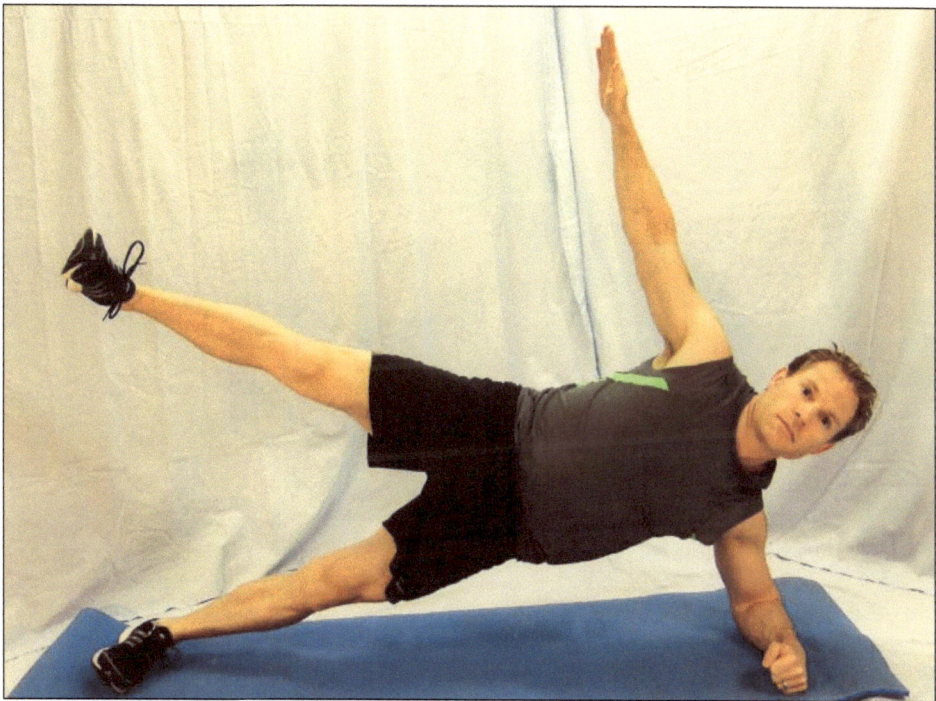

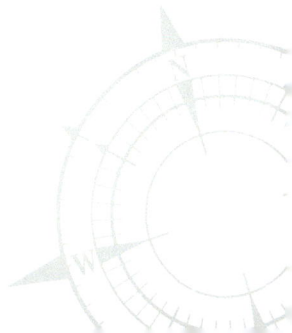

*"CONFIDENCE WILL MAKE
YOU DARING"*

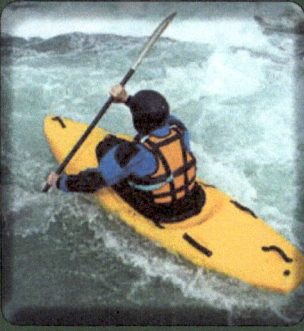

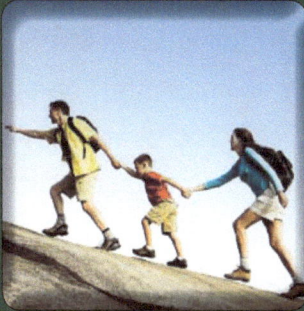

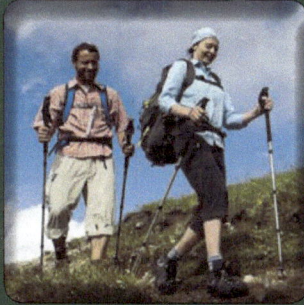

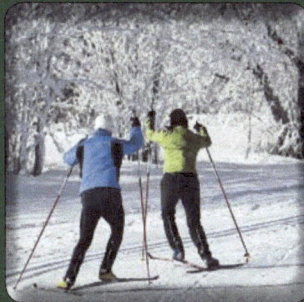

CHAPTER 6:
COORDINATION, BALANCE, AGILITY, & BODY AWARENESS

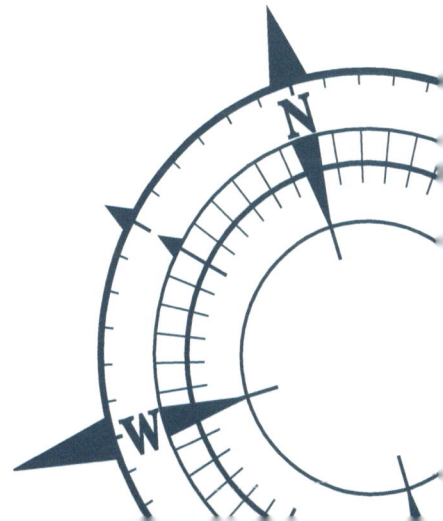

For most of my clients, the most rapid progress in functional fitness occurs in the areas of coordination, balance, and agility. Improvement is often seen from the first to the second set the first time they perform an exercise. Equally important is that the functional fitness gained in these fitness components transfers very easily and noticeably to everyday activities and recreational endeavors.

I postulate that this rapid improvement occurs for three major reasons. The first is that coordination, balance, and agility are woefully under-trained and underdeveloped in most individuals. Many traditionally "fit" individuals don't employ enough activities that benefit these components because the majority of the exercises they use are linear and artificially stabilized (think of the machine circuit at any health club).

The second reason I think rapid improvement occurs is that we all grew up running, skipping, jumping, throwing, and climbing. Playground activities and exploring the woods, streams, and fields all rely on and develop balance, coordination, and agility. The point is that our bodies know how to do these things. At some point, most of us "grew up" and we just stopped doing them. Thus, it is not much of a stretch to challenge our body to relearn some of these skills.

The final reason rapid improvement occurs is that these exercises are fun. Clients love doing them.

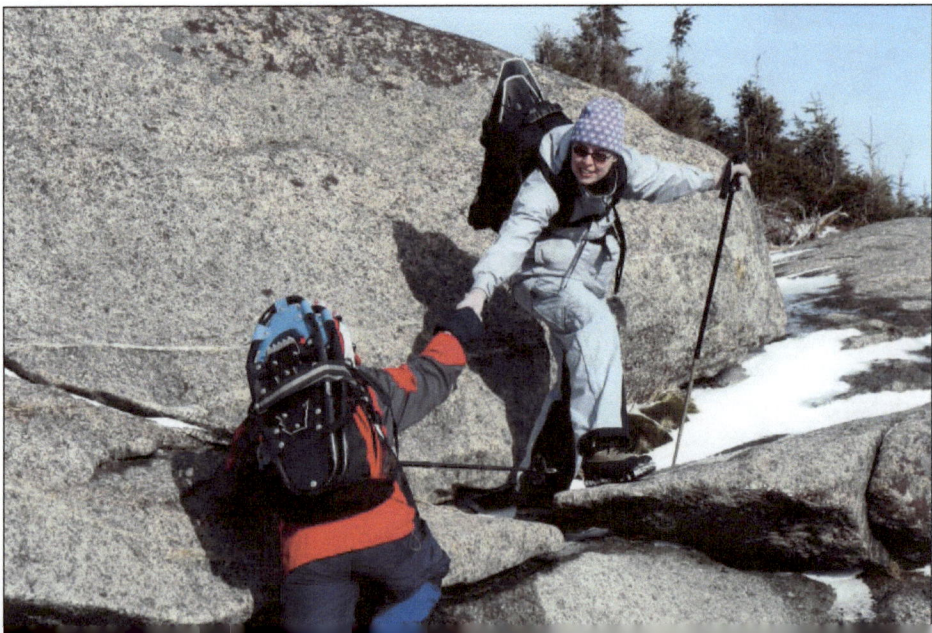

Another very significant result of training the functional fitness components of coordination, balance, and agility is the kinesthetic awareness that you develop. Simply put, you become consciously and subconsciously aware of where your body and its various parts are in relation to each other and the world around you. This gained body awareness is an almost spiritual revelation to many under-trained individuals and is invaluable in its own right. But, of equal significance is that this kinesthetic awareness makes you much more capable of dealing with the unexpected—the loose rock on the hiking trail, the dog that cuts in front of you while running, the moose that you find as you come around a corner on a ski trail…. You are better prepared for the surprises life throws at you.

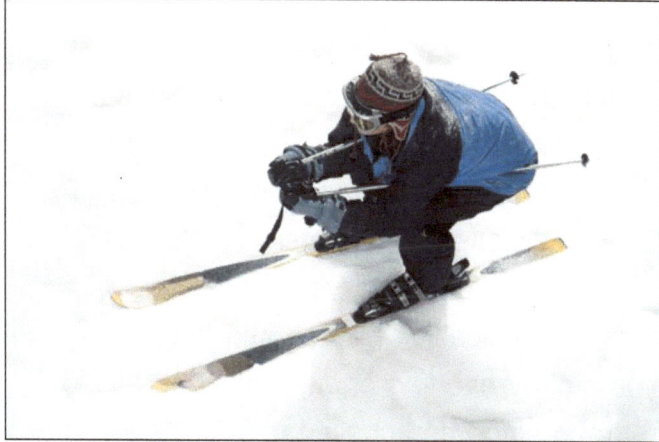

Your performance in many outdoor activities is at its best when you execute them aggressively at the edge of your abilities, particularly activities such as skiing or mountain running. By increasing your functional capacity in the areas of balance, coordination, and agility, you can significantly expand your capabilities. Improved kinesthetic awareness leads to confidence and confidence will make you daring.

The following are several dynamic exercises that will significantly improve your coordination, balance, and agility. In addition, these movements are demonstrated in the video clinic on dynamic movements at www.spartanfitnessalaska.com.

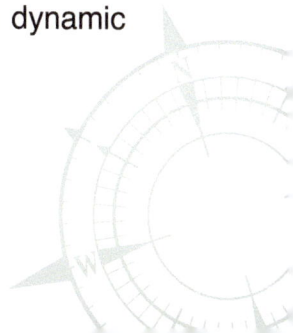

SPEED SKATERS

You can perform speed skaters with your body weight or with a medicine ball. Effective, quick, and controlled transfer of body weight from one foot to another, not only in the forward plane but in the lateral plane as well, is a fundamental skill required in virtually any athletic activity. Stride from side to side, emulating the movement seen by speed skaters or skate skiers. You want to keep your head up, your body low, and move athletically. You should challenge yourself by exerting enough effort to allow a broad stride and challenge your balance by spending significant time on one foot and gaining control of the outward momentum you've generated.

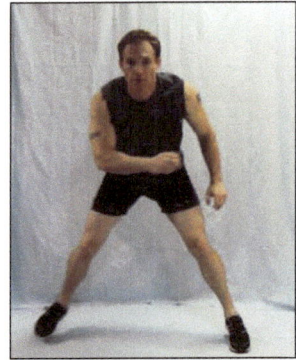

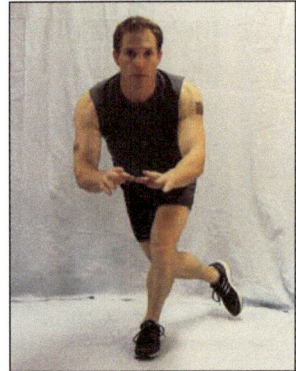

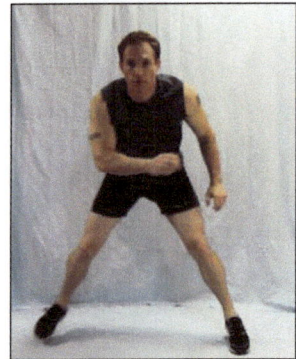

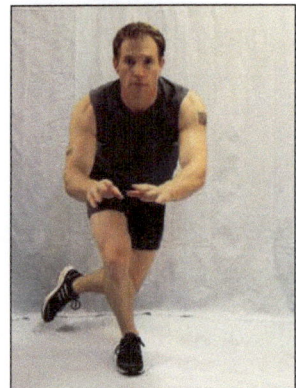

JUMPS

Jumping is a very natural and functional movement that can be performed in a wide variety of ways to develop power, balance, and agility. This activity develops explosive leg strength and power that can be utilized when climbing, bouldering, or biking. In addition to the strength developed in the jump, the landing develops balance and coordination. Single leg jumps further these capacities and replicate practical movements like stream crossings.

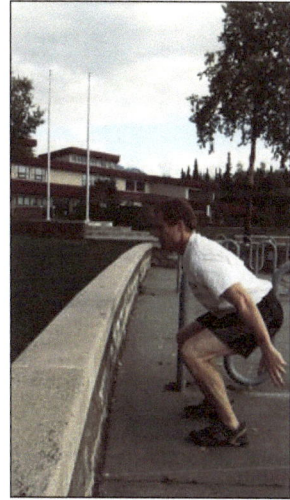

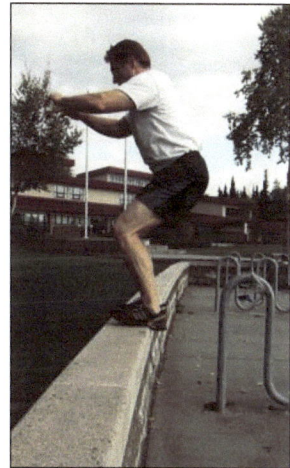

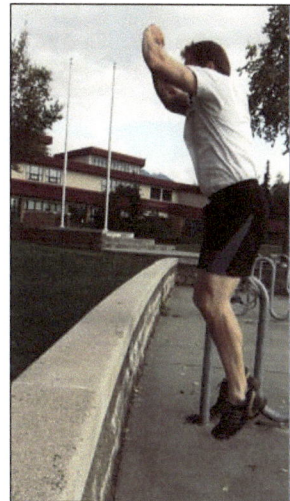

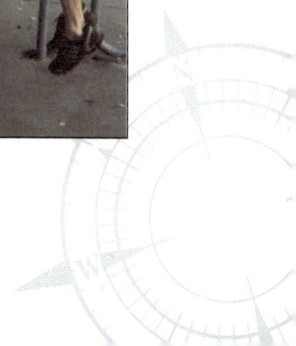

SINGLE LEG HOPS

This exercise will develop balance and develop the stabilizing muscles of the lower leg. Many athletic endeavors ranging from ice skating to skate skiing to running require that significant time be spent on a single foot. If you are stable on one foot, you will be rock solid on two feet. Single leg hops should be performed forward and backward as well as side to side.

FRONT TO BACK

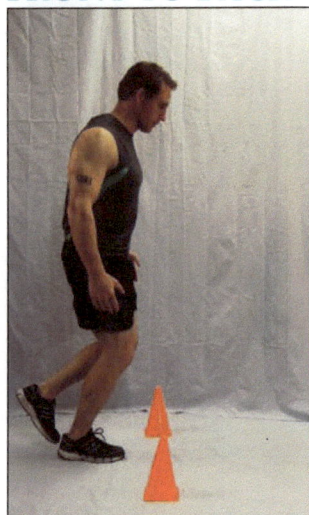
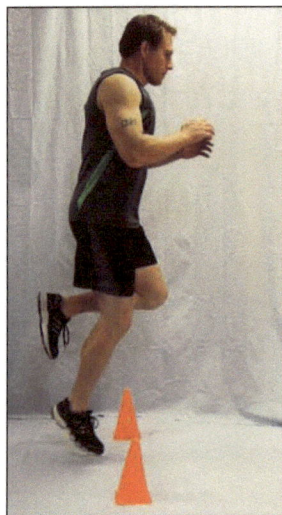
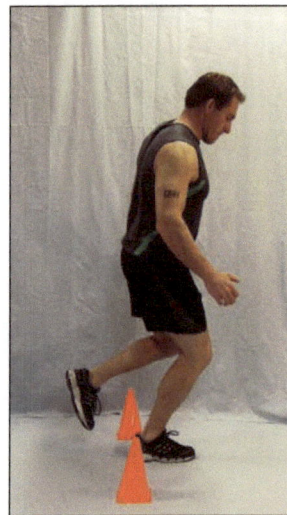

SIDE TO SIDE

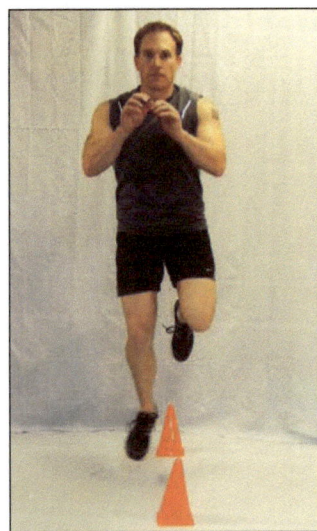
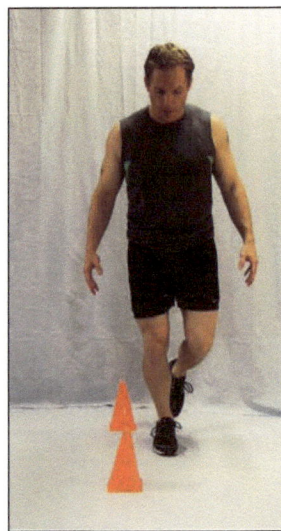
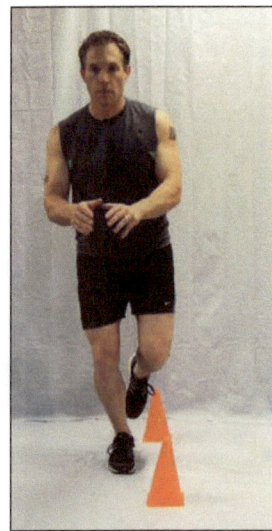

LEG ABDUCTIONS AND ADDUCTIONS

These exercises enhance balance and strengthen the muscles of the inner and outer thighs, hips, and lower leg. Stand on one leg and raise the other leg to the side and away from your body (abduction) while keeping your knee straight. Similarly, remain standing on the same leg and raise the other leg up and across your body (adduction) as high as possible while keeping your leg straight. The higher you lift your leg, the greater the effort of the hip muscles and challenge to your balance.

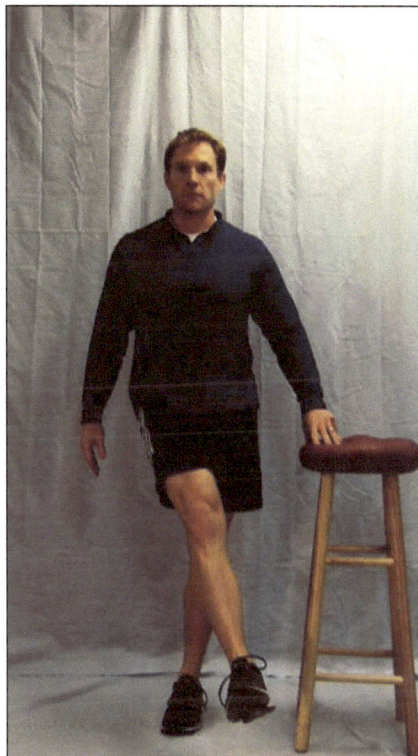

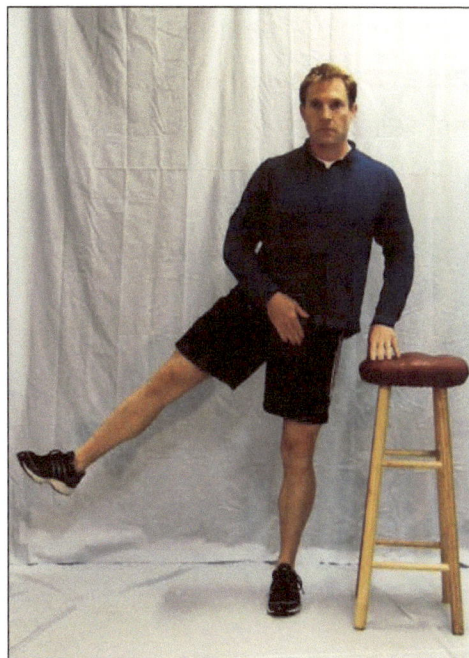

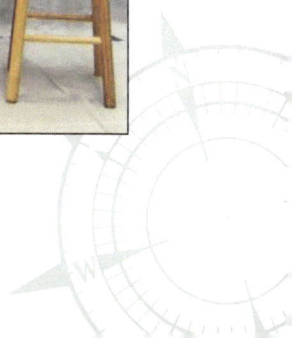

MEDICINE BALL TOE TAPS

This exercise is very effective at developing quick feet, balance, and coordination. Your goal is to tap the top of the ball with alternate feet as quickly as you can. Start slowly and build up speed as your balance allows. You should keep your eyes on the ball throughout the exercise, as it can roll. The quick foot movement, agility, and accurate foot placement are essential to activities like mountain running, particularly on the descent. In addition to developing agility, medicine ball toe taps require significant oxygen and thus provide metabolic benefit as well.

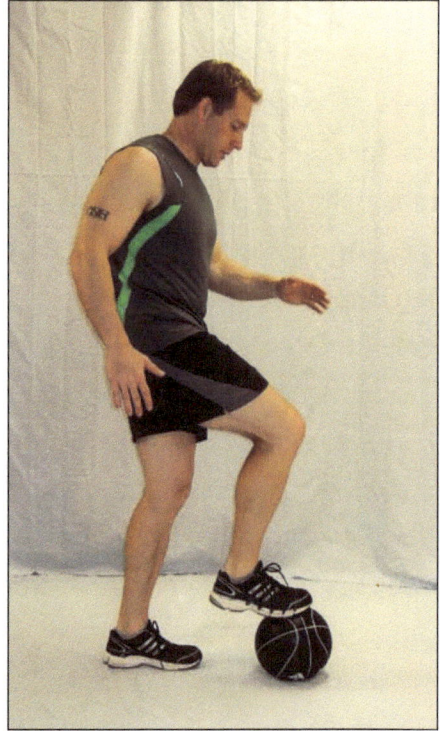

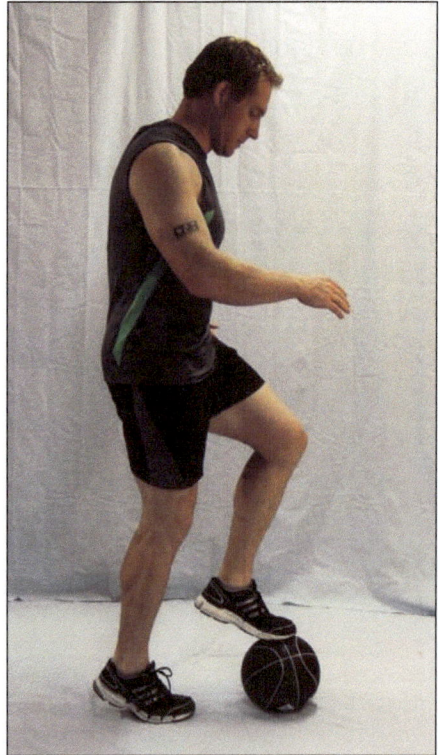

SWING KICKS

Swing kicks develop coordination by requiring body control in both the forward and lateral planes. Significant time is spent on one leg, thus enhancing balance. Further, the hip flexors are fully engaged throughout the movement. The combination of balance and high stepping has practical applications when climbing and bouldering. Hip flexor power and muscular endurance benefit the hip rotation and kick utilized in many common swimming strokes.

RIGHT LEG

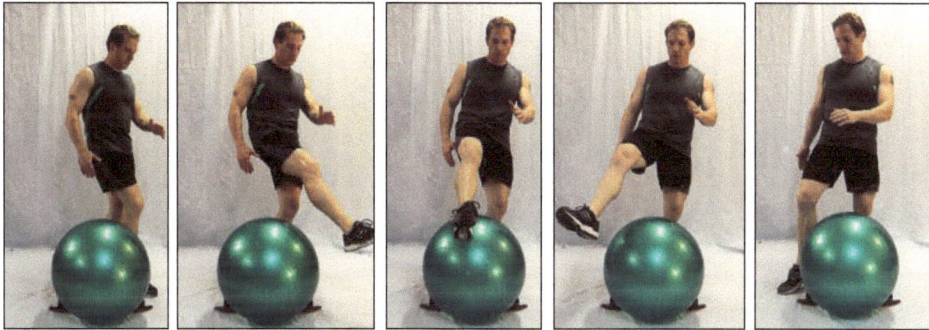

LEFT LEG

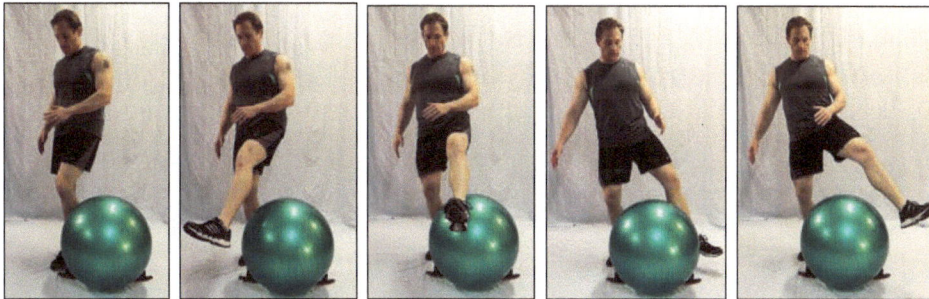

STEP UPS – FORWARD AND SIDE TO SIDE

Step ups develop foot speed, agility, and coordination. These exercises have obvious applications for activities including hiking, climbing, and trail running. However, active and agile footwork are critical for other endeavors such as skiing and skating.

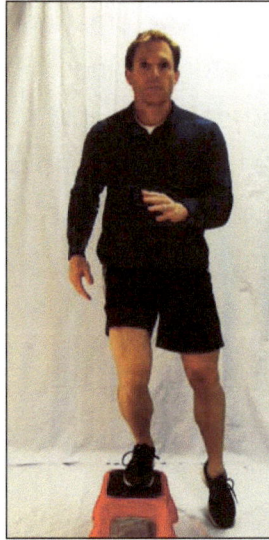

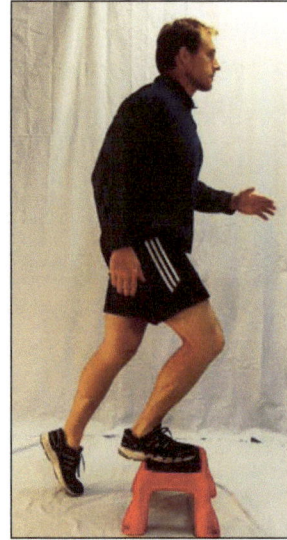

Step ups should be performed forwards and backwards as well as side to side. Increase speed or step height to increase metabolic intensity and further challenge your balance.

CALF LEANS

Many athletic activities ranging from running (particularly downhill) and skiing require an aggressive forward stride or stance. Calf leans enhance your ability to control your body weight in a forward leaning posture. Further, they fully engage all of the muscles of the lower leg. To perform this exercise, lean forward as far as you can (imagine you are ski jumping). You want to find the edge of your balance where you are just barely in control and hold this position. Be sure to stand near a wall or other sup-

portive structure so you can prevent a full fall forward.

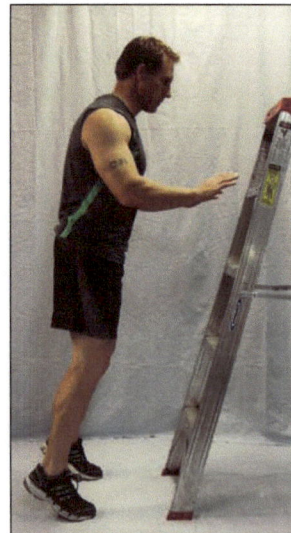

AGILITY RUNS

We want to be proficient not only in the forward plane, but also the lateral plane. Sideways runs and shuffles engage the lateral muscles of the upper thigh and the muscles of the lower leg. This has practical benefits when hiking or running on undulating trails of varied terrain or performing activities that utilize significant lateral movement such as ice skating, skate skiing, or rollerblading. In addition, this activity enhances agility and coordination. When performing these exercises, keep your head up, your butt down, and your feet quick.

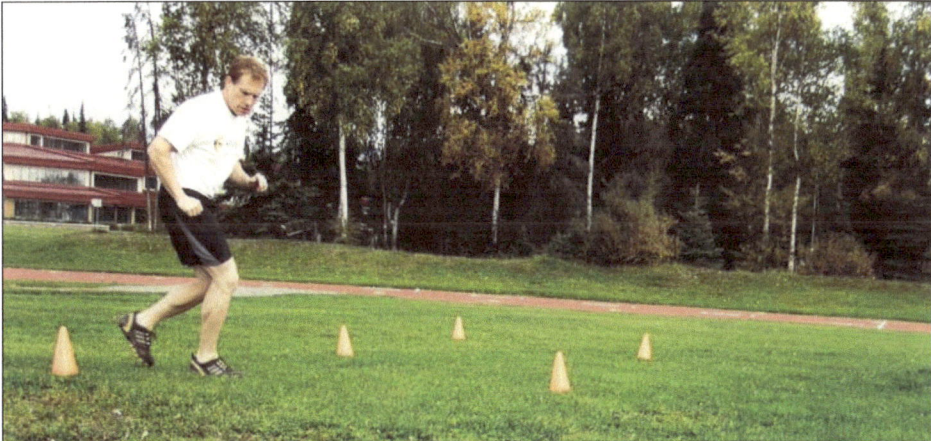

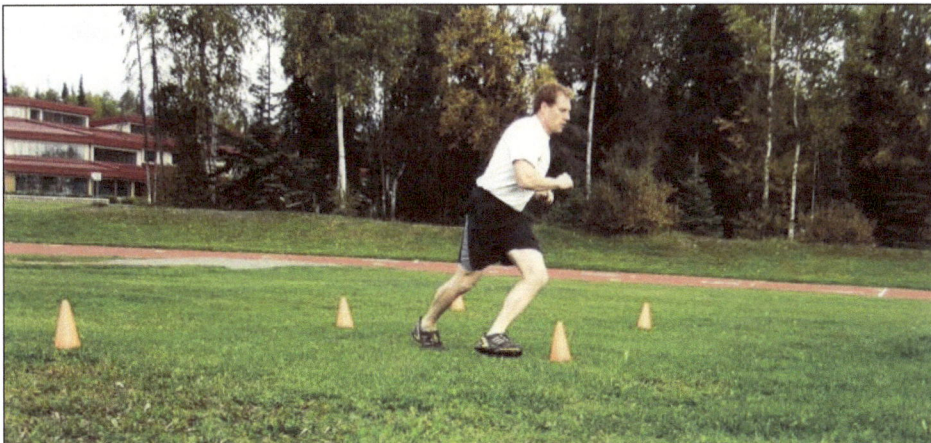

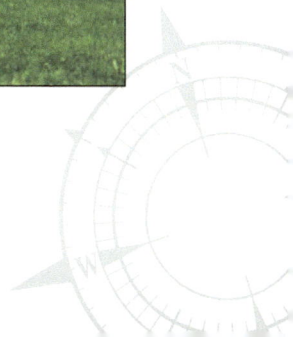

MEDICINE BALL WALL TOSSES

Medicine ball wall tosses are simply a thruster where the ball is launched upward and then caught as it returns earthward. Similar to thrusters, this exercise enhances one's ability to generate and transfer power from the legs to the upper body and overhead. Medicine ball wall tosses also challenge one's focus and coordination.

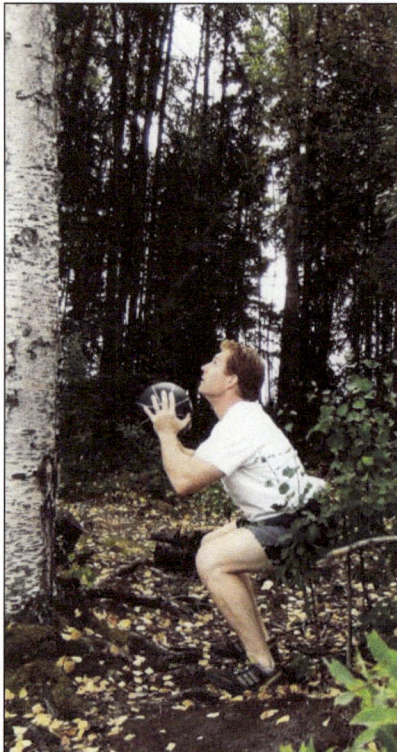

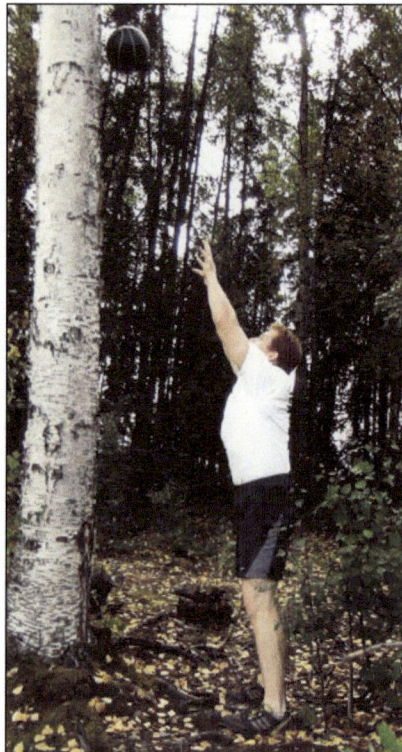

ROPE AND WALL CLIMBING

Rope climbing, when performed correctly, is an outstanding full-body movement that requires significant coordination. Ensure that your climbing environment is safe.

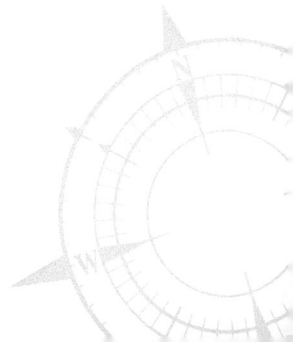

*"YOU CAN PRODUCE MORE POWER
BY MOVING YOUR MUSCLES
AND JOINTS THROUGH THEIR
FULL RANGE OF MOTION"*

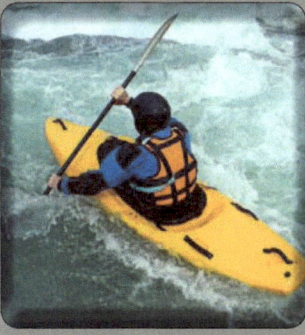

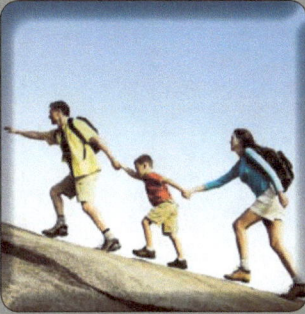

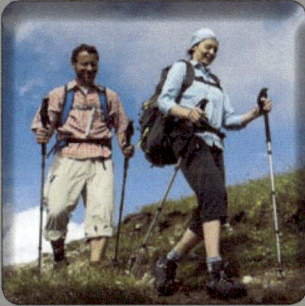

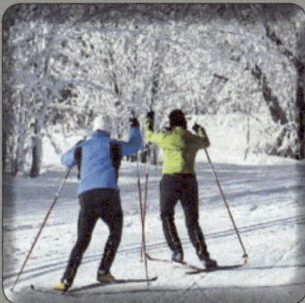

CHAPTER 7:
FLEXIBILITY &
RANGE OF MOTION

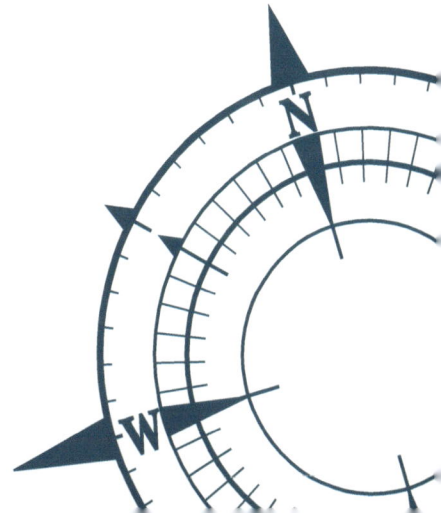

Flexibility is the elasticity of an individual muscle group (e.g., the hamstrings) and range of motion is the multiplanar movement potential across a joint. These two components of fitness are critical to all aspects of physical performance. Similar to balance and agility, these aspects are often significantly under-trained. The benefits of increased flexibility and range of motion are twofold. The first is that risk of injury is reduced when you encounter activities at the edge of your abilities. The second is that you can produce more power

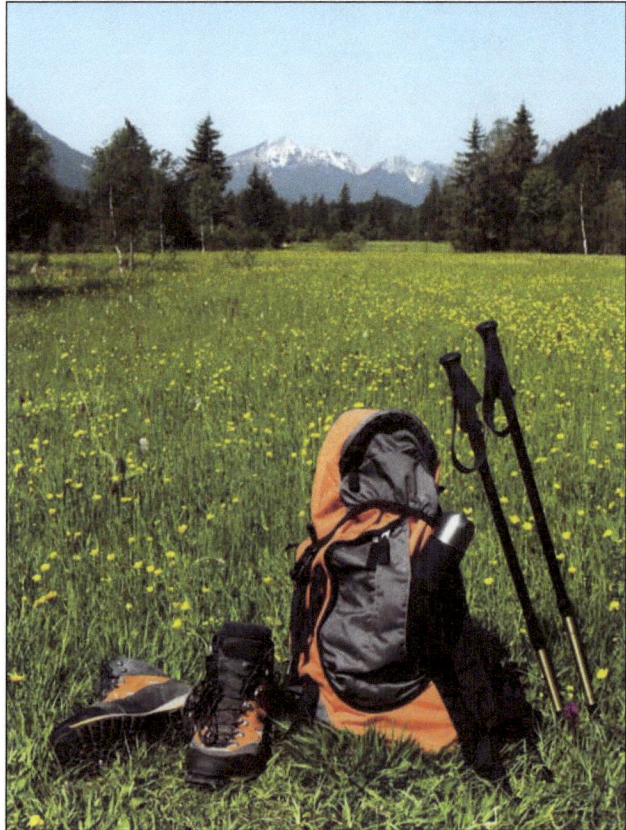

by moving your muscles through their full range of motion. Utilizing the full range of motion across joints is like removing the resistors from an electrical circuit. The net result is greater energy and power delivery. This principle applies to any physical activity, from rowing to climbing to skiing to biking. Significant performance improvements can be gained by fully utilizing the mechanical advantages available from the hips, hamstrings, and shoulder girdle. Further, the risk of common injuries can simultaneously be prevented.

There are two primary and complementary ways that flexibility and range of motion can be dramatically improved. The first is performing all of the activities described in previous chapters through their full range of motion. As one example, it is generally not advisable to do deep squats (i.e., where the hips drop well below the knee) with an external load. However, body weight or light weight squats can be done as deep as your body allows and range of motion can improve with practice through time. Recognize that billions of humans throughout the world eat, pray, converse, and relieve themselves in a deep squat, even at advanced ages.

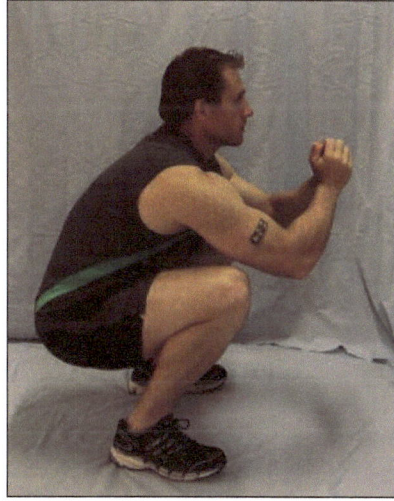

The second way to improve flexibility and range of motion is through deliberate stretching exercises. As in the chapters above, there are a seemingly endless number of stretches one can perform to improve flexibility and range of motion. In addition, certain forms of exercise include a primary focus on these fitness components (e.g., yoga, Pilates). The following are a few basic stretches that address the primary muscle groups and joints of the body. For further guidance, visit www. spartanfitnessalaska.com.

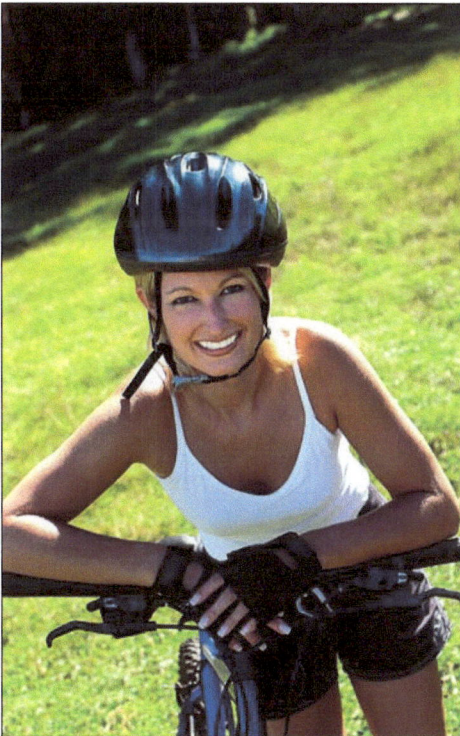

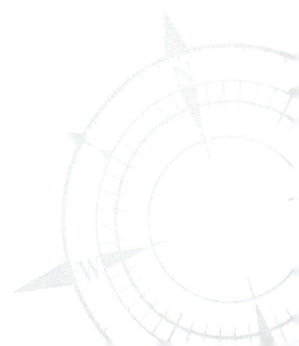

GROIN AND INNER THIGH

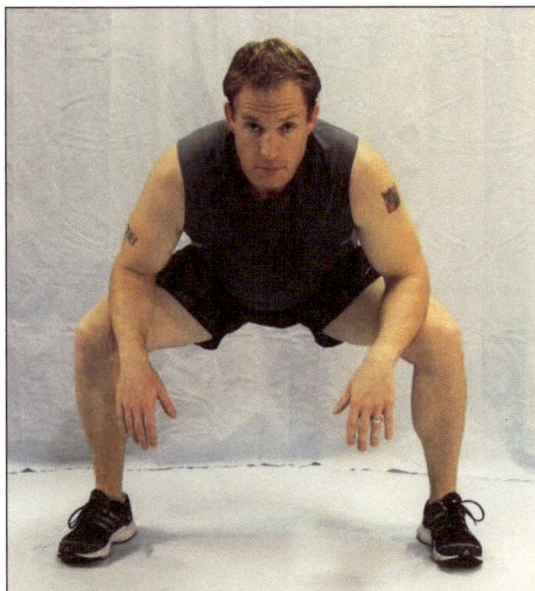

To stretch the groin and inner thigh, drop into a wide, deep squat. Using your elbows for leverage, slowly and gently open your knees wider to stretch the inner thigh.

HAMSTRINGS

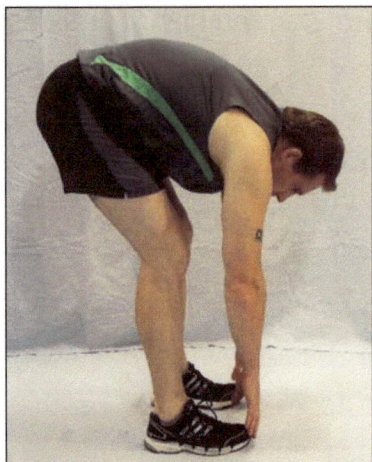

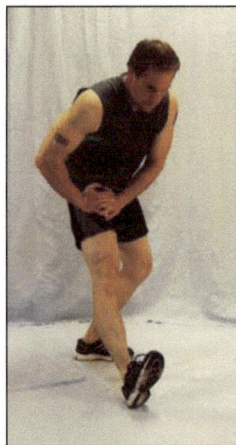

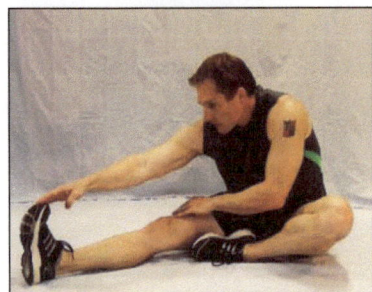

Tight hamstrings are common in many individuals. Thus, particular attention should be paid to this muscle group. The hamstrings can be stretched in an upright standing, bent over, or sitting position. Regardless of the position you choose, you want to gently place and hold tension on the hamstrings. Each of these variations will also stretch the lower back.

HIP FLEXORS

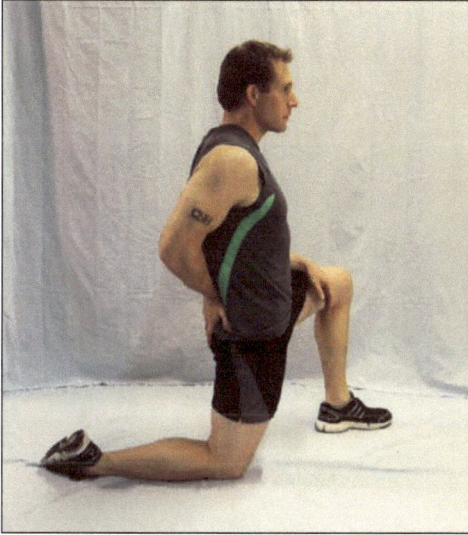

To stretch the hip flexors, kneel on one knee and roll your hips forward. You can aid this stretch by pushing on your rump to further your hip from behind.

QUADRICEPS

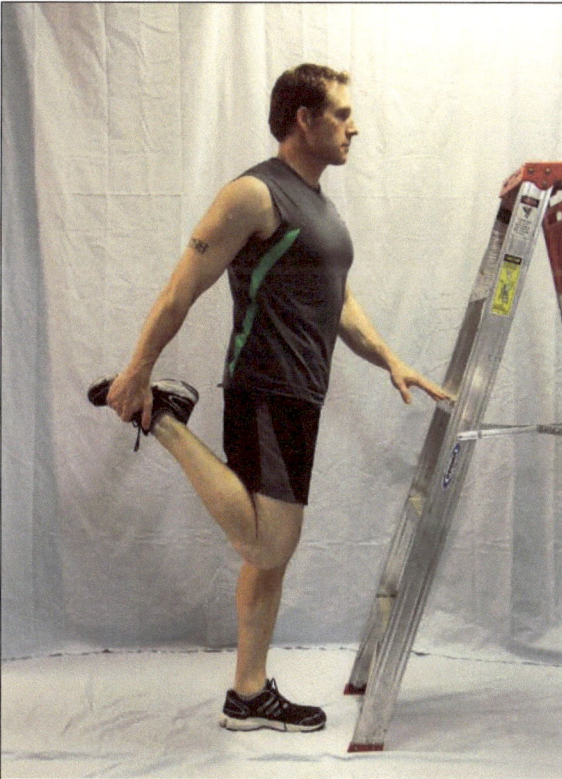

The quadriceps are best stretched from a standing position. Grasp the front of your foot just below the ankle and slowly and gently apply force to stretch the quadriceps muscle group. Ensure you have a wall or other object available to assist your balance.

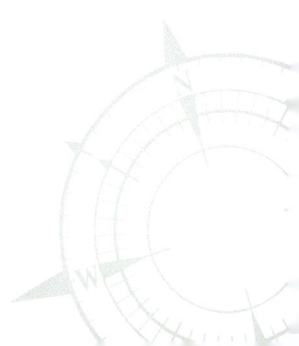

CALVES

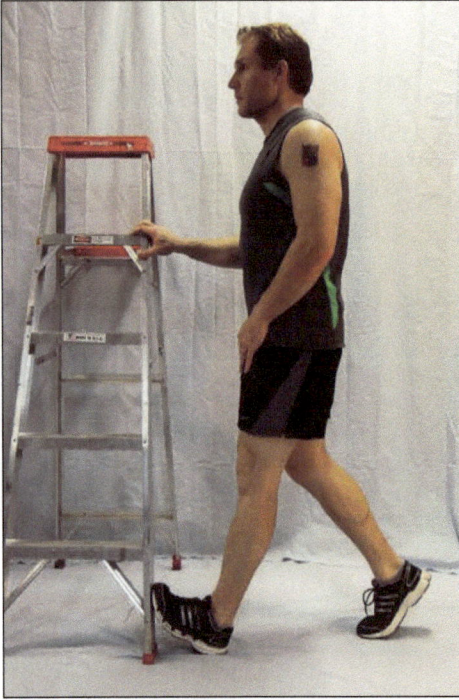

The calves can be stretched by placing your toes against a wall and heel on the floor forming a roughly 45° angle between your foot and the floor. Keeping your leg straight, slowly press your body towards the wall with your other foot and leg.

SHOULDERS

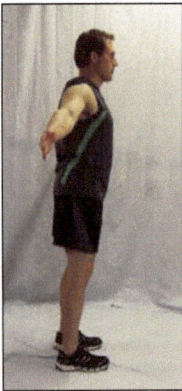

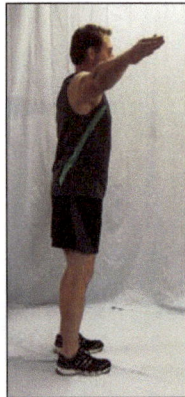

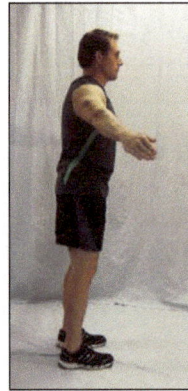

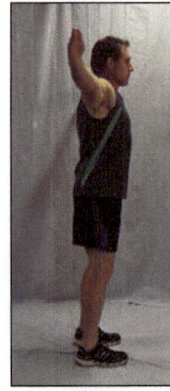

To improve flexibility in the shoulder girdle, hold your arms directly away from your body as if forming the shape of a cross. Begin rotating your arms forward forming small circles with your hands and slowly increase the size of the circle until you are at your full range of motion in the shoulder joint. Repeat this movement, but in the reverse direction.

CHEST

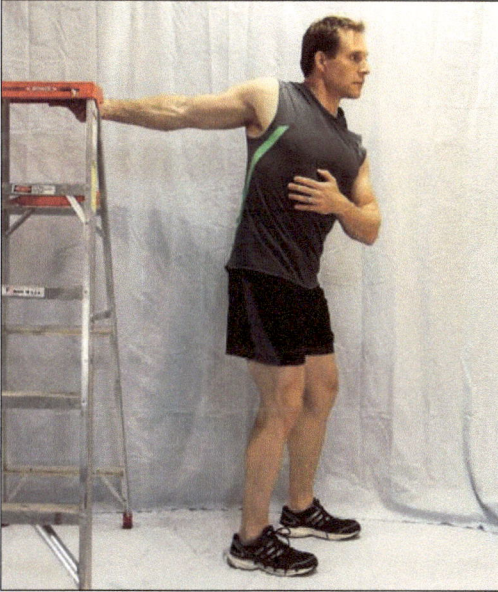

The chest can be stretched effectively by placing your hand on a static object such as a pole or wall. Simply rotate you body away from this object to open your chest and your body weight will provide the force producing the stretch.

BACK

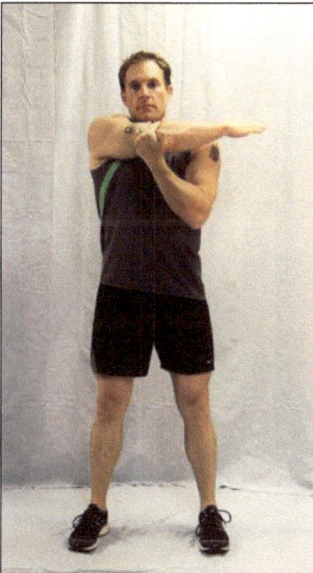

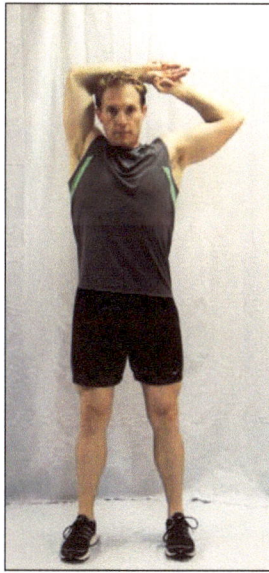

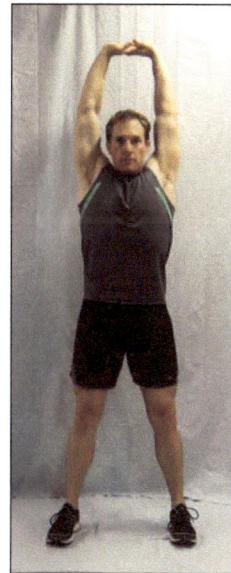

To stretch your back, use the leverage available in your arms by pulling each arm across and above your body. Also, interlock your fingers and reach fully over head to stretch your spinal muscles.

NECK

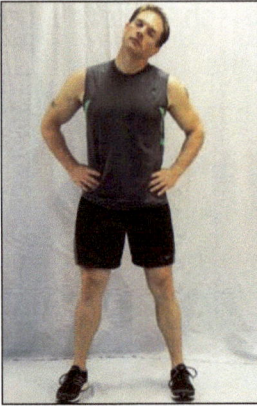

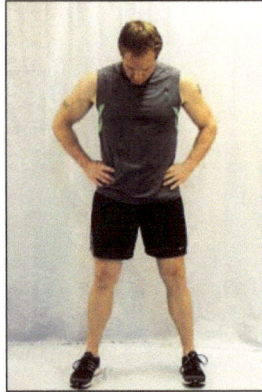

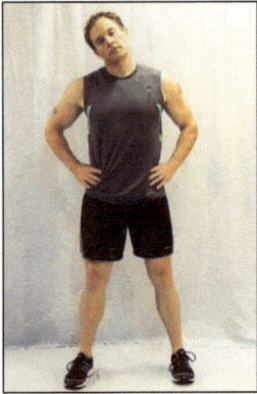

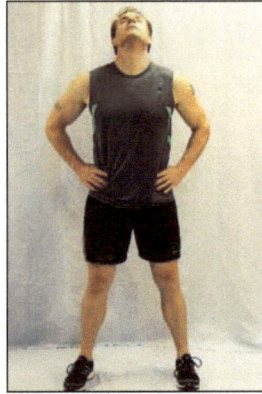

The warm up and stretch the neck, simply roll your head slowly and deliberately several times clockwise. Repeat the movement in the opposite direction.

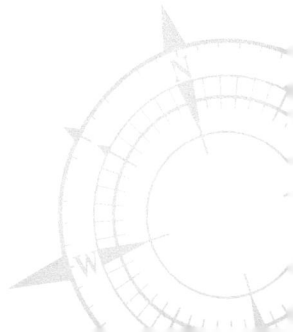

"ENGAGING IN NEW ACTIVITES
CHALLENGES YOUR FITNESS
IN NOVEL WAYS"

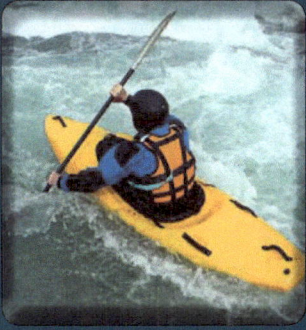

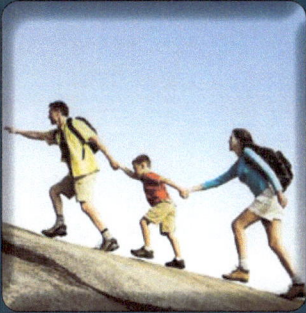

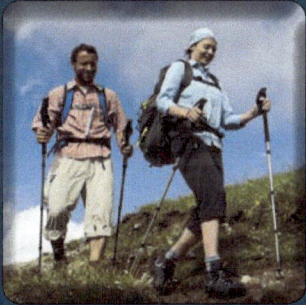

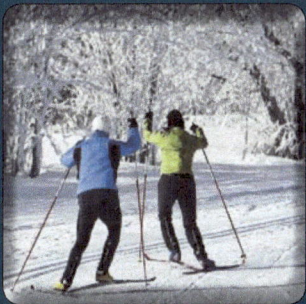

CHAPTER 8:
RECREATION AS TRAINING

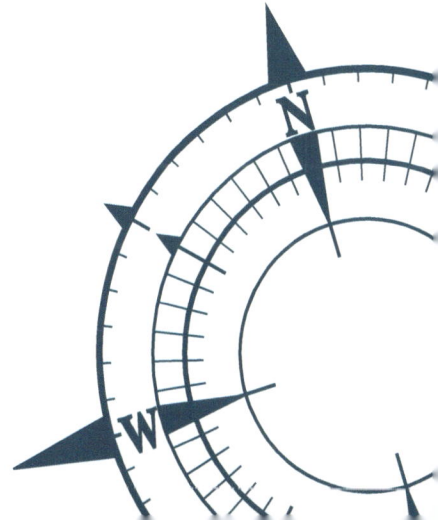

Running, biking, swimming, hiking, climbing, skiing, canoeing, and kayaking can all provide multiple benefits across the fitness components addressed in the preceding chapters. As functional movements, they inherently benefit functional fitness. These enjoyable activities can provide diversity, both physical and mental, to workout programming, and the practice of a variety of activities allows you to train throughout the year regardless of the climate you live in.

While there is obvious benefit to participating in these activities purely for their enjoyment, a different mindset is needed when engaging in these pursuits as part of a program with the intent of improving overall performance. Crossfit® has developed the useful mantra of "constantly varied, high intensity, functional movement" that serves us well when using recreational activities to benefit functional fitness.

Include variation in your program not only by performing multiple activities such as biking, running, and swimming, but by varying your approach within a specific activity. For example, conduct long, relatively slow runs on trails with varying terrain that includes uphill and downhill segments. It is beneficial to focus on goals of either time or distance in long duration, low intensity sessions. Balance these sessions with other sessions that include shorter duration, higher speed segments (e.g., 400 m sprints conducted in a circuit with pushups and medicine ball cleans). Further, you can instill variation within a given session of a given activity. When running along a road, walk from the first light pole to the second, jog to the third, sprint to the fourth, and repeat. Alternatively, walk for a minute, jog for a minute, and run for a minute, and repeat. In essence, we are including periodization and interval training across and within workouts, respectively.

To ensure intensity, monitor your heart rate and time. Watches or wrist bands that include both a timer and a heart rate monitor can be purchased at most sporting goods stores. Timing your activities will provide an accurate assessment of your progression through time. In addition, competing with the clock naturally motivates most individuals.

Below is a chart identifying target heart rates for individuals by age. As previously mentioned, ensure you have consulted with your physician and that these targets are appropriate for you.

Age (years)	Target Heart Rate* (beats per minute)
<20	100-170
25	98-166
30	95-162
35	93-157
40	90-153
45	88-149
50	85-145
55	83-140
60	80-136
65	78-132
>70	75-128

*range from 50% to 85% of maximum heart rate

By monitoring both time and heart rate during the course of your activities, you will stay mentally engaged. One of the problems with running on the treadmill at the gym is that many folks are lulled by the television or other distractions. They end up going through the motions. While any physical activity has benefits, distracted efforts minimize gains, reduce efficiency, and dampen the mind-body connection we are striving for.

Finally, look to learn new activities. This will allow you to be active throughout the year and the benefits of developing new skills and training new motor pathways will further utilize and enhance your kinesthetic awareness. Also, don't be afraid to hire a coach or take some lessons.

I grew up largely in the flatlands of the Midwest. The first (and what I expected would be the last) time I downhill skied I was about sixteen. Some friends and I traveled to Lake Benton, Minnesota, to a small ski hill. I slapped on some poorly fitted skis, clutched the rope that served as the ski lift, and was towed stumbling to the crest of the hill, where I promptly crouched into my Olympic tuck. (I only knew what I had seen on TV ...remember the "agony of defeat" video clip from ABC's Wide World of Sports.) It never dawned on me to ask anyone how to stop....I guess I thought it would come naturally. I made six runs down the mountain that day, each of which ended in me basically bailing to one side or the other at about thirty miles per hour to avoid running into the chalet. After each catastrophic ending, I would collect my scattered hat, gloves, skis, and poles and start over again (that was the day I learned the phrase "yard sale"). My knees, wrists, and back were sore for a week and my pride for even longer.

In my early thirties, my wife, who grew up skiing in the Alps, enrolled our three-year-old daughter in downhill lessons. Every Saturday, she would spend two hours skiing with an instructor and a group of about six other kids and rapidly became proficient. Growing somewhat envious of the fun she was having and growing restless just sitting around and waiting, I decided I may as well give it another try. This time, however, a little wiser and with a little more disposable income, I took a few lessons. What a difference! Within fifteen minutes I was comfortable and understood how to use my body effectively to manage my balance and control my momentum. Today, skiing with my daughter is one of my absolute favorite activities. It is so much more rewarding than sitting on the sidelines watching. Thankfully, she graciously allows me to catch up every now and then.

The key is that my level of functional fitness gave me the confidence to try and the capacity to succeed at learning a new skill relatively quickly. Engaging in new activities challenges your fitness in novel ways and requires a heightened coordination between your mind and your body. Thus, look for new activities to try and seek guidance from enthusiastic experts who enjoy teaching. Don't be bashful about finding a trainer or coach, or joining a class or club (e.g., Nordic ski club, crew team, trail running association). These activities can then serve as a source of year-round recreational enjoyment and offer new and challenging training opportunities.

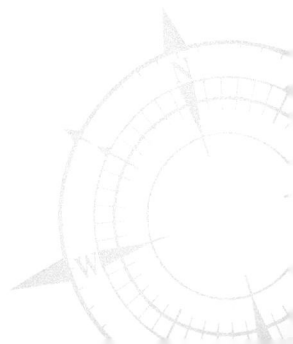

*"PROGRAMMING IS HOW
WE TURN A PILE OF STONES
INTO A CATHEDRAL"*

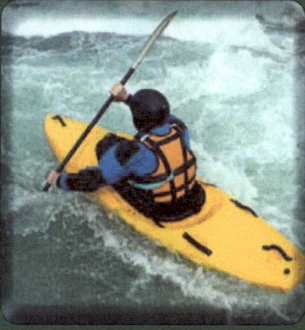

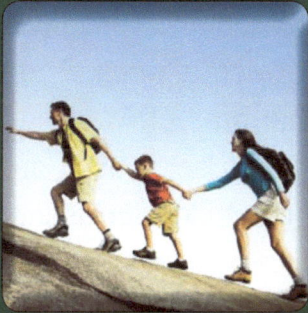

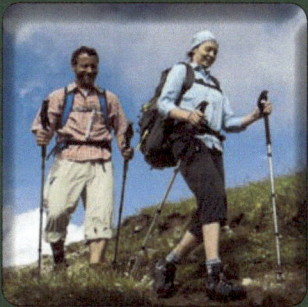

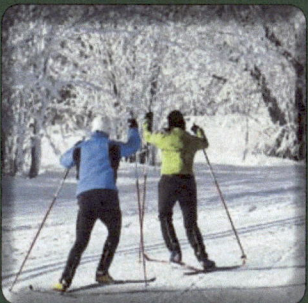

CHAPTER 9:
PROGRAMMING – PUTTING IT ALL TOGETHER

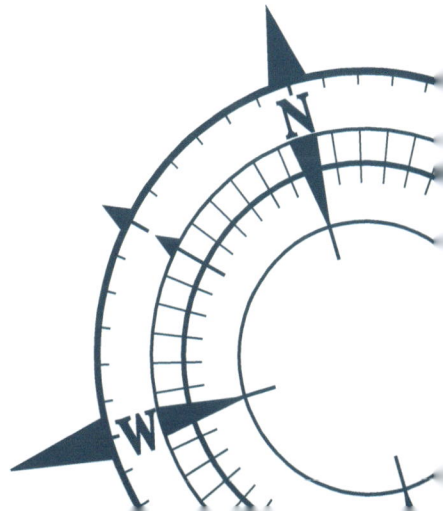

Programming is how we put together all of the pieces described in the previous chapters. It is how we develop a truly integrated fitness that forms our mosaic of power, endurance, flexibility, and kinesthetic awareness. It is how we turn a pile of stones into a cathedral.

I think this is the most important chapter in the book. In many ways, it is the simplest. In many ways, it is the most complex. The one message I want to convey to readers is that "routine" is to be avoided. From age 14-30 I used one of the more common and generic workout routines. I would go to the gym every Monday, Tuesday, Thursday, and Friday working each body part twice a week. The common lingo among my gym mates was "what are you working today," to which the appropriate response was "legs," or "back," or "chest." These simple one word answers carried with them significant meaning met with a detailed understanding that "chest" most likely included some mix of bench press, dumbbell flies, cable crossovers, and the like. This weight work was then followed by a 30–60 minute session on a treadmill, elliptical, or stationary bike.

Not only were my metabolic pathways (aerobic and anaerobic) and fitness components (muscular strength and cardiovascular endurance) compartmentalized and trained separately, even my individual muscle groups were further divided, treated so independently that I worked them on separate days. How can this be the best approach to developing functional fitness across a variety of activities in a wide range of environments? It is not an organic approach.

I don't want to imply that all of my time training in this manner was wasted (or, if this routine type of training sounds familiar to you, that your time was entirely wasted, either). In fact, it did provide me with a significant foundation of strength and cardiovascular endurance. However, my efforts were not as efficient or as transferable to the world outside the gym as they could have been.

Instead, what I argue we should strive for is constant variation in exercises, order, intensity, and execution. Look to structure workout sessions that emphasize both balance and unpredictability. Also, develop skills in a variety of seasonal activities that will allow you to include recreation as part of your training program throughout the year. This approach will consistently stimulate your body to adapt and increase the fitness components discussed in previous chapters. Further, it will avoid the mental boredom and fatigue that come with over-structured and repeated routines. Finally, the varied approach will lead to a high level of year-round functional fitness that will translate well to the variety of physical activities in which you, as an outdoor recreation generalist, joyfully participate.

As examples, I have listed fifteen days of workouts for two of my clients. One is an advanced client who trains five to six days per week and the second is an intermediate client who works out three to five days per week. These examples are not meant to be routines to be followed. Rather my intent in presenting them is to illustrate the blending of the different fitness components and the variation that occurs from one workout to the next.

CLIENT 1 (ADVANCED):

Day 1

Warm up and stretching

Circuit 1: Squats (heavy) – 5 sets of 8–12 repetitions

Pull-ups – 5 sets of 8–15 repetitions

Dips – 5 sets of 12–20 repetitions

Circuit 2: Anchored abdominal raises – 3 sets of 12–15 repetitions

Lying back extensions – 3 sets of 60 seconds

180° Surfers – 3 sets of 30 repetitions

Medicine ball toe taps – 3 sets of 100 taps

Stretching

Day 2

Warm up and stretching

Circuit 1: Dead lifts (heavy) – 5 sets of 8–12 repetitions

Decline bench press (heavy) – 5 sets of 6–12 repetitions

Shoulder press – 5 sets of 8–12 repetitions

Circuit 2: Abdominal raises – 3 sets of 12 repetitions

Bird dogs – 3 sets of 60 seconds

Single leg hops (forward and back, side to side) – 3 sets of 5 repetitions

Swing kicks – 3 sets of 12 cycles

Stretching

Day 3

2 hour hike, 1500 ft. elevation gain

Day 4

Rest

Day 5

Warm up and stretching

Circuit 1: Thrusters – 4 sets of 12–15 repetitions

Rows (heavy) – 4 sets of 8–12 repetitions

Pushups – 4 sets of 12–20 repetitions

Circuit 2: Planks – 3 sets of 30–45 seconds

Calf leans – 3 sets of 30 seconds

Jumps – 3 sets of 15 repetitions

Stretching

Day 6

Warm up and stretching

Test day – for time:

¼ mile run, 20 squats (body weight), 12 dips

¼ mile run, 20 squats (body weight), 12 dips

¼ mile run, 20 squats (body weight), 12 dips

¼ mile run

Stretching

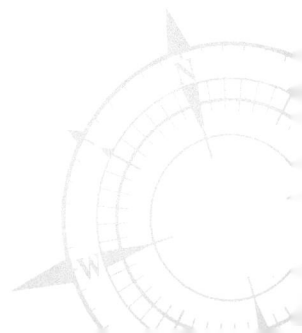

Day 7

Warm up and stretching

Circuit 1: Power cleans – 4 sets of 8–12 repetitions

Bicep curls – 4 sets of 8–15 *(okay ...sometimes I yield to vanity—he has a class reunion approaching)*

Calf raises – 4 sets of 12–20 repetitions

Circuit 2: Moth to cocoons – 3 sets of 15 repetitions

Bird dogs – 3 sets of 60 seconds

Speed skaters – 3 sets of 45 seconds

Medicine ball wall toss – 3 sets of 15 repetitions

Stretching

Day 8

Rest

Day 9

Warm up and stretching

For time:

7 medicine ball cleans, 7 pushups, ¼-mile run

7 medicine ball cleans, 7 pushups, ½-mile run

7 medicine ball cleans, 7 pushups, ¾-mile run

7 medicine ball cleans, 7 pushups, 1-mile run

Flexibility work

Stretching

Day 10

Warm up and stretching

Circuit 1: Dead lifts to upright rows – 5 sets of 12 repetitions

Push presses – 5 sets of 8–12 repetitions

Rows – 5 sets of 8–12 repetitions

Circuit 2: Bicycles – 3 sets of 12–15 repetitions

Straight leg dead lifts – 3 sets of 12 repetitions

80:20 squats – 3 sets of 12 repetitions with each leg

Agility runs – 3 sets of 4 laps

Stretching

Day 11

15 mile bike ride

Day 12

Rest

Day 13

Warm up and stretching

Circuit 1: Power cleans (moderate) – 5 sets of 8–10 repetitions

Pull-ups – 5 sets of 8–15 repetitions

Shoulder presses – 5 sets of 8–12 repetitions

Circuit 2: Lunges – 3 sets of 15 repetitions with each leg

Step ups (forward, backward, and sideways) – 3 sets of 45 seconds

Planks (front and side) – 3 sets of 30–60 seconds

Stretching

Day 14

Warm up and stretching

Squats (body weight) – 20 seconds on, 10 second rest, for 4 minutes

Pushups – 20 seconds on, 10 second rest, for 4 minutes

3 mile jog

Stretching

Day 15

5 hour hike, 3500 feet elevation gain

CLIENT 2 (INTERMEDIATE):

Day 1

Warm up and stretching

Circuit 1: Squats (moderate weight) – 3 sets of 12 repetitions

Pushups – 3 sets of 12 repetitions

Calf leans – 3 sets of 30 seconds

Rows – 3 sets of 12 repetitions

Circuit 2: Medicine ball toe taps – 3 sets of 80 taps

Planks – 3 sets for 30 seconds

Agility runs – 3 sets of 3 laps

Stretching

Day 2

Rest

Day 3

Warm up and stretching

Circuit 1: Thrusters – 3 sets of 10–15 repetitions

Assisted pull-ups – 3 sets of 12 repetitions

Assisted dips – 3 sets of 12 repetitions

Circuit 2: Sideways step ups – 3 sets of 30 seconds

Moth to cocoons – 3 sets of 12 repetitions

Bird dogs – 3 sets of 60 seconds

Stretching

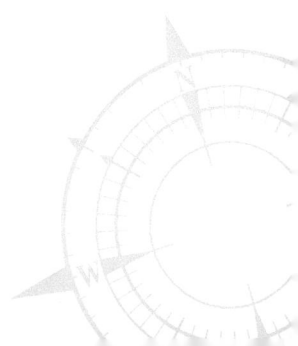

Day 4

Rest

Day 5 - Outside in local park

Warm up and stretching

Circuit 1: Lunges – 3 sets of 10–15 repetitions

Medicine ball cleans – 3 sets of 10–12 repetitions

Shoulder presses – 3 sets of 12–15 repetitions

Circuit 2: Speed skaters – 3 sets of 45 seconds

Anchored abdominal raises – 3 sets of 12 repetitions

Lying back extensions – 3 sets of 60 seconds

180° surfers – 3 sets of 30 repetitions

Stretching

Day 6

Outdoor activities on own – 90 minute bike ride

Day 7

Rest

Day 8

Warm up and stretching

Circuit 1: Dead lifts – 4 sets of 12–15 repetitions

Push presses – 4 sets of 10–12 repetitions

Assisted pull-ups – 4 sets of 12–15 repetitions

Circuit 2: Jumps – 3 sets of 12 repetitions

Swing kicks – 3 sets of 12 cycles

Straight leg dead lifts – 3 sets of 12–15 repetitions

Bicycles – 3 sets of 12–15 repetitions

Stretching

Day 9

Rest

Day 10

Warm up and stretching

Circuit 1: Body weight squats – 8 sets of 15

Pushups – 8 sets of 10

Circuit 2: Agility runs – 3 sets of 3 laps

Single leg hops (forward and back, side to side)
– 3 sets of 5 repetitions

Circuit 3: Abdominal raises – 3 sets of 12–15 repetitions

Bird dogs – 3 sets of 60 seconds

Shoulder flexibility

Stretching

Day 11

Rest

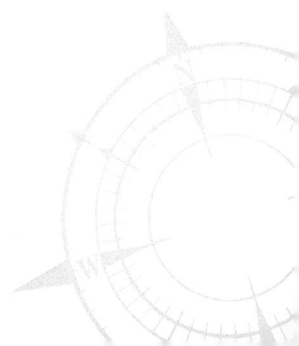

Day 12 - Outside in local park

Warm up and stretching

Circuit 1: Cleans with medicine ball – 3 sets of 10–12 repetitions

Abductions and adductions – 3 sets of 15 repetitions

Shoulder press – 3 sets of 10–15 repetitions

Upright rows – 3 sets of 10–12 repetitions

Circuit 2: 80:20 squats – 3 sets of 12 repetitions per leg

Planks – 3 sets of 30 seconds

Stretching

Day 13

Rest

Day 14

Outdoor activity on own — 1 hour hike

Day 15

Warm up and stretching

Circuit 1: Dead lifts to upright rows – 5 sets of 12–15 repetitions

Bench press – 5 sets of 10–12 repetitions

2 mile run

Circuit 2: Bicycles – 3 sets of 12–15 repetitions

Birddogs – 3 sets of 60 seconds

Stretching

As you look over these two programs, several patterns should emerge. The first is that, while there is little repetition of exercises and no repeated routines, many of the workouts contain full-body resistance movements that span numerous joints and require the control of an external object (e.g., barbell, dumbbell, or medicine ball). These full-body movements certainly require and develop muscle and bone strength. The recruitment of several large muscle groups, requires significant oxygen to meet metabolic demands, thus both the aerobic and anaerobic pathways are utilized and trained. Further, due to the need to generate and control the transfer of momentum from one part of the body to another (generally, large muscles to smaller muscles), the core is actively engaged as a stabilizer and significant balance is required. Finally, by performing these movements through their full range of motion, flexibility is enhanced.

A second pattern is the inclusion of heavy weight work such as barbell squats, dead lifts, and bench press, as well as lighter weight resistance work using one's body weight or a medicine ball. The heavy load work requires significant effort over a shorter duration, thus focusing on the anaerobic metabolic pathways. The lighter load work can be performed at an increased pace per repetition or for a longer duration. This approach will focus on muscular endurance and providing both aerobic and anaerobic benefits.

A third pattern to note is that many of the resistance exercises are performed in a circuit. This allows reduced downtime, as one muscle group is recovering while another is being trained. The overall intensity can be managed through the amount of rest between sets of exercises. This approach elevates heart rate throughout the resistance portion of the workout, thus blurring the line between "weights" and "cardio". This decompartmentalization is both efficient and practical.

A fourth pattern is a crafted balance in the selection of the resistance exercises such that a "push" exercise is balanced with a "pull" exercise. For example, pull-ups may be paired with dips. This is directly counter to the compartmental approach of "back" days and "chest" days. In essence, within any given workout, most of the body is actively engaged at one point or another.

A fifth pattern is the frequent and specific inclusion of exercises that explicitly challenge one's balance, coordination, and agility. Almost every client I have worked with has been largely undertrained in these components of fitness. However, this is the training area where they have seen the most dramatic improvement, the most practical transferability outside the gym, and identify as the most fun. An additional benefit of this work is that, if performed at high intensity with limited rest, cardiovascular endurance can be enhanced. Perhaps the most compelling reason to train for balance, coordination, and agility is their direct link to one's physical confidence. My clients have quickly changed their mindset relative to certain activities from "I can't do that" to "I'll give it a try" to "let's do it again, only higher or faster."

A sixth pattern is the prescription for warming up and stretching before and after each session. This helps prepare the body for the work ahead by elevating body temperature and increasing heart rate. Most importantly, the pre-workout stretch, in concert with proper form, can prevent muscle, ligament, or tendon injuries. The post-workout stretch, coupled with exercises performed through a full range of motion, will improve flexibility.

A seventh pattern is the inclusion of rest days. Rest means rest. Take it easy. Your body needs to recuperate and recharge periodically.

A final pattern is the occasional timed workout that serves to set benchmarks and monitor achievement through time by assessing performance across the majority of the fitness categories.

When approached this way, it is obvious that a limitless number of workouts can be crafted. The art lies in constructing workouts that are constantly varied and span the categories of fitness widely. The science requires that the exercises are balanced, performed at high intensity, and include warm ups and stretching each session.

*"YOUR BODY IS DESIGNED
TO HANDLE AND UTILIZE
HIGH QUALITY, NUTRITIOUS,
WHOLE FOODS"*

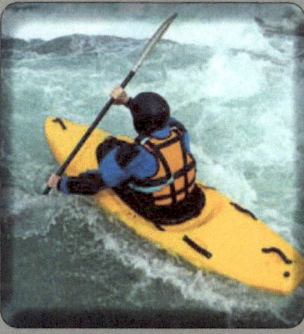

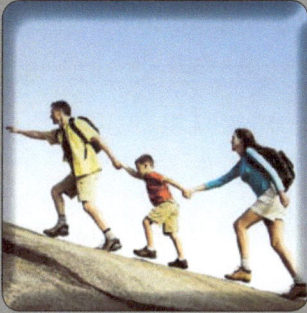

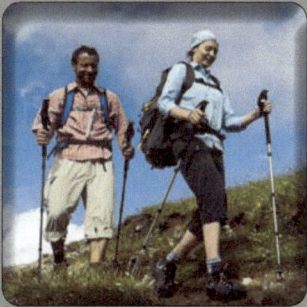

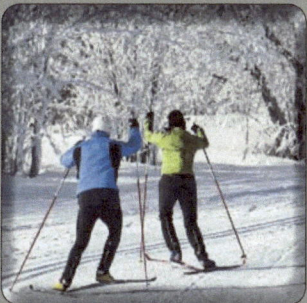

CHAPTER 10:
NUTRITION

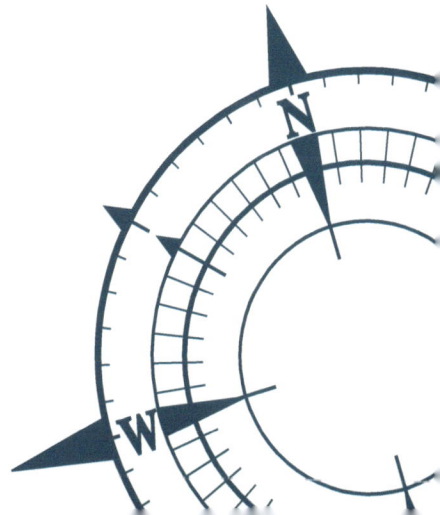

It seems impossible to write a book on fitness without dedi-
cating some print to the topic of nutrition. After all, the nutrients we
ingest are the building blocks that are key to maintaining our bodies,
supporting tissue growth, and fueling the energetic demands of our
activities. However, few topics have been more over-hyped, over-
analyzed, and over-exploited than nutrition.

I provide my clients with a one page handout that summarizes
about 95% of what you need to know relative to nutrition to maximize
your fitness. My intent is to simplify the chaotic multitude of mes-
sages that barrage all of us relative to the latest approach or newest
fad. That handout is the foundation of this chapter and is organized
into the following general rules:

Rule 1: Diets don't work. You need to develop good habits,
meaning choices you can repeat every day for the rest of
your life.

Rule 2: Quantity. Don't eat more than your body needs.
Don't own huge plates. Get "normal" plates. Don't fill your
plate (leave some white space) when serving. Take a
twenty minute break before going for seconds to ensure
that you are truly hungry. If you do take seconds, take 1/3
of your original serving.

Rule 3a: Quality. Fresh, local foods are best, followed by
frozen, then canned.

Rule 3b: Quality. Whole foods are better
than processed foods. If you have a choice,
select whole grain breads, pastas, and rice.

Rule 3c: Quality. Choose color. Pick red,
green, yellow, and orange vegetables over
white carbohydrates like potatoes or rice.

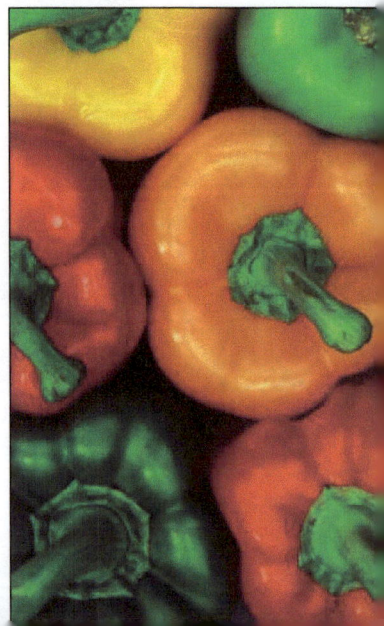

Rule 3d: Quality. Shop the outside aisles of the grocery store first. This is where the perishable and, thus, most nutritious items are located (e.g., fresh fruits and vegetables, meat and eggs, fresh whole grain breads, and dairy items). The center aisles typically contain items with a long shelf life (i.e., those which contain significant amounts of preservatives). By starting on the outside aisles of the store, you won't over-purchase since the foods will spoil. If you enter the store hungry, your impulse buys will be healthier.

Rule 4: Eat consciously. Don't eat while watching TV, surfing the Internet, driving, reading a book, etc. Learn your body's cues regarding satiation and follow them. Eating consciously will also allow you to pay attention to flavor. You will find that your body truly prefers high quality, fresher foods.

Rule 5: Moderation. Completely giving up sugar, caffeine, or alcohol is a noble pursuit but is unrealistic for many. The cravings lead to binging which leads to guilt. Allow for some consumption of these items but strive for moderation.

Rule 6: Don't fear fats. Quality fats such as those found in vegetables, fish, olive oil, and nuts are vital to proper body function. Avoid "fat-free" foods as this doesn't necessarily mean low calories—often these items are very high in processed sugars.

Rule 7: Your body needs protein. Protein can be acquired through a wide variety of sources including meat and eggs, dairy products, nuts, and vegetables. When selecting meats, pay attention to portion size, cut, and type. Don't

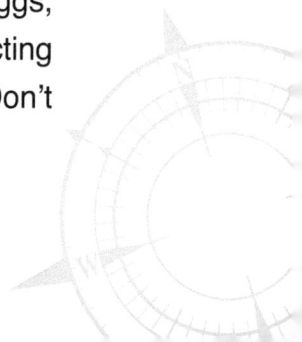

short your body on this important nutrient, especially when in training (which is all the time, right?).

Rule 8: Hydrate, hydrate, hydrate. You are an ocean surrounded by skin. Adequate hydration is critical to proper organ function, metabolic processes, and physical performance.

Rule 9: Awareness. Consider keeping a food journal. This will help make you aware of the decisions you are making. Strive to make at least one decision you are proud of each day.

Rule 10: Plan ahead. Limited options lead to poor decisions.

Rule 11: Avoid fast food. Even if you walk in the door planning on a salad, there is too much temptation (see Rule 10). I am not against burgers. Just eat a good one made with fresh, high quality ingredients. The best way to ensure this is to make it yourself.

Rule 12: Spread your calories out during the day. Consuming five to six small meals rather than three large ones will help regulate your insulin and blood sugar levels. This will benefit your mental and physical performance.

Rule 13: Don't beat yourself up, don't stress, and don't obsess.

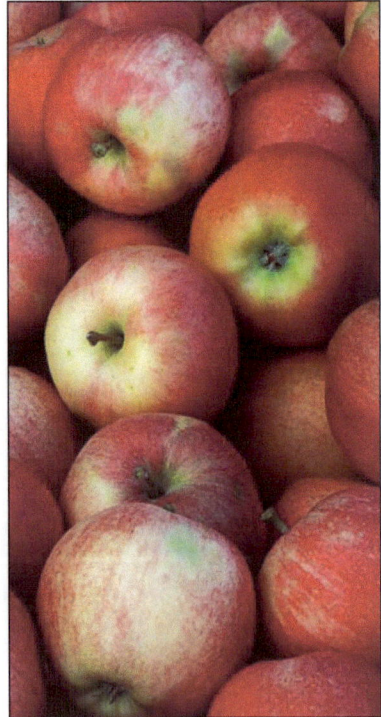

What is in the past is the past. It is like Karma. Move forward and strive for your good decisions to outweigh your poor ones.

Rule 14: Enjoy food! Food is your friend, not the enemy. It is important that you mantain a positive relationship with what you eat.

My experience has been that as people improve the quality of the food they consume, their cravings change also. The high sugar, highly processed, and preservative-laden foods lose much of their appeal. Your body is designed to handle and utilize high quality, nutritious, whole foods. As your diet improves, your mental function will be keener and your physical performance more dynamic. More than anything, you will simply feel better, less bloated, and cleaner due to a more natural water balance and reduced levels of superfluous additives and preservatives.

Finally, your body requires water and energy to perform effectively and recover adequately. You need to ingest quality calories roughly ninety minutes to an hour prior to strenuous exercise and thirty to sixty minutes following exercise. Additionally, when enjoying outdoor activities, be sure to carry ample water and food to ensure adequate hydration and to meet energy demands.

*"KNOWLEDGE AND PREPARATION
ARE THE KEYS"*

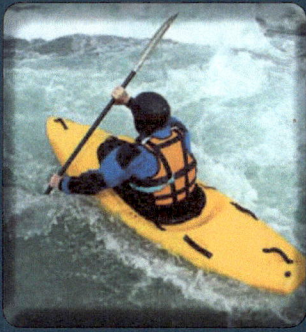

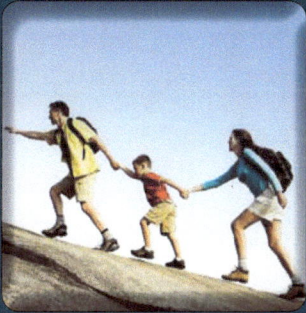

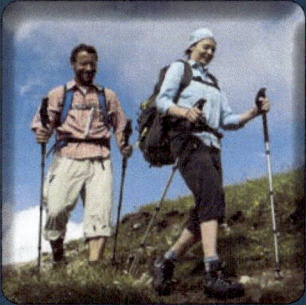

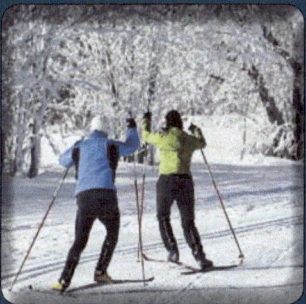

CHAPTER 11:
THE ELEMENTS

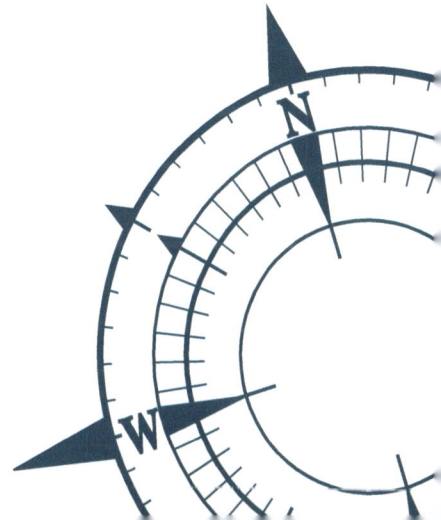

The primary intent of this book is to provide you with a foundation of fitness to allow you to fully enjoy life and the great outdoors. Keep the following factors in mind to minimize the likelihood of minor inconveniences and major injuries when heading outside for training or recreation.

Weather: Be aware of the sun, the wind, and the rain. Carry and use sun block of appropriate strength as well as sunglasses to protect your skin and eyes. Clothes are also important tools that can prevent hypothermia by minimizing heat loss due to cold temperatures, wind, or precipitation. Similarly, appropriate clothing can help prevent hyperthermia by allowing heat and moisture transfer through the fabric. Some fabrics offer UV protection as well.

Bugs and plants: Be knowledgeable of local insects and plants, particularly if you have allergies. Don't eat any wild plant unless you are sure you can accurately identify it and know it is safe to consume. Bug repellent and a head net can really come in handy so keep them in your pack.

Animals: In some regions, moose, bears, snakes, and other wildlife reside where we love to recreate. The key is to stay alert and make noise. If you see an animal, give it a wide berth or, if necessary, reverse your direction. Most negative encounters result from surprising an animal or approaching too closely.

Training: Consider taking a first aid class and stay current on your CPR certification. In addition, many areas offer wilderness first

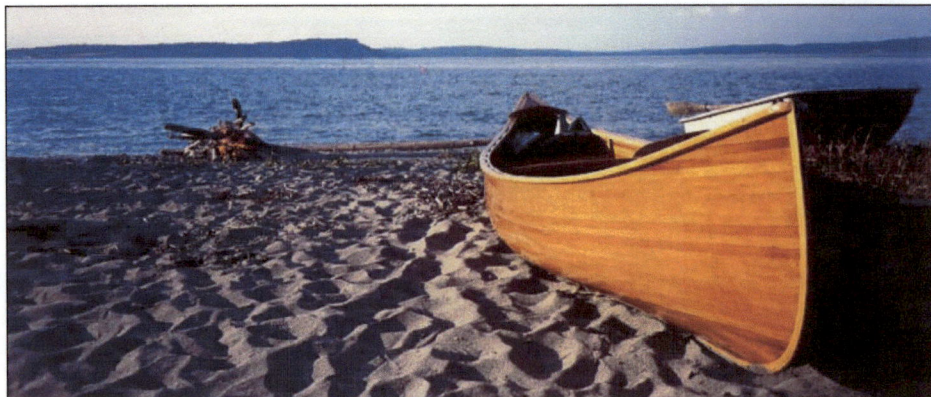

aid courses. In the event of an emergency, knowledge and preparation are the keys to survival.

First aid kit: If you are getting off the pavement, compile a first aid kit and keep it with you.

Share your plan: Tell someone where you are going and when you plan to return.

Snow: If you are engaging in winter activities off groomed trails, consider taking a course on snow and avalanche safety or obtaining a guide book on assessing snow conditions.

Map, compass, and/or GPS: Getting lost can ruin your day. Carry the right tools and learn how to use them. Besides, orienteering is a fun way to utilize your functional fitness.

Footgear: Take care of your feet. My experience is that good shoes are a great investment. Use the right shoes with the right tread for the activities you are engaging in. Further, go to a store that knows how to fit and outfit you properly. Socks are also important. Synthetics will protect your feet from blisters and keep you warmer than cotton. In cold weather, wool can be the right option.

Food and water: Take more than you need. Also, for remote activities, carry a water filtration system or purification tablets in your pack.

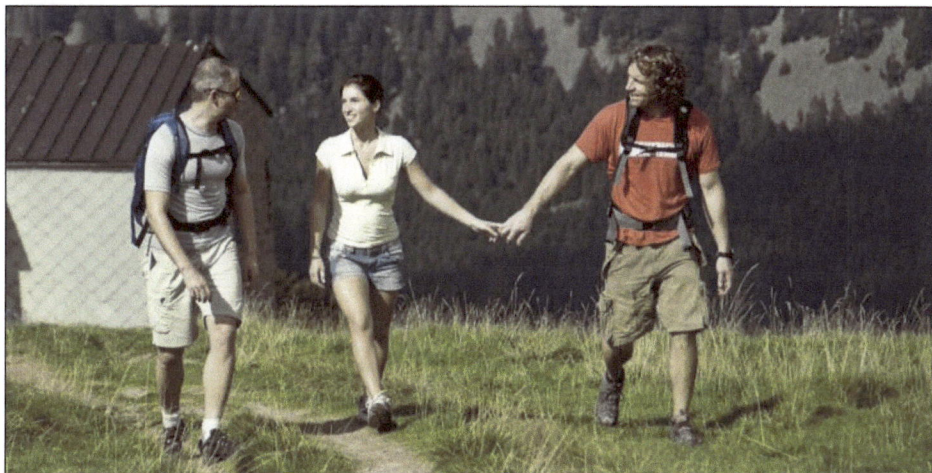

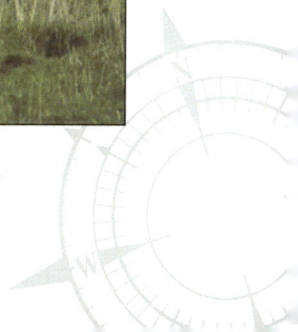

"ENJOY YOUR JOURNEY"

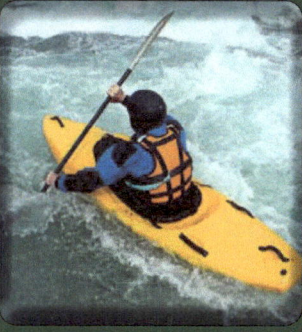

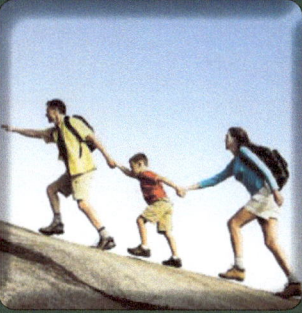

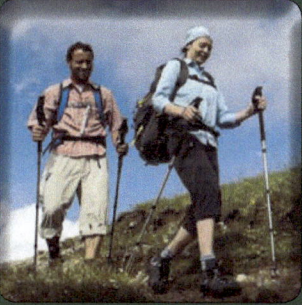

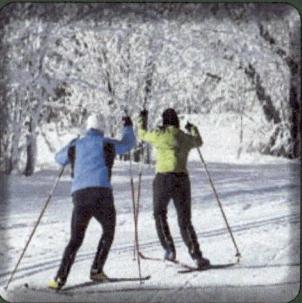

CHAPTER 12:
SYNTHESIS

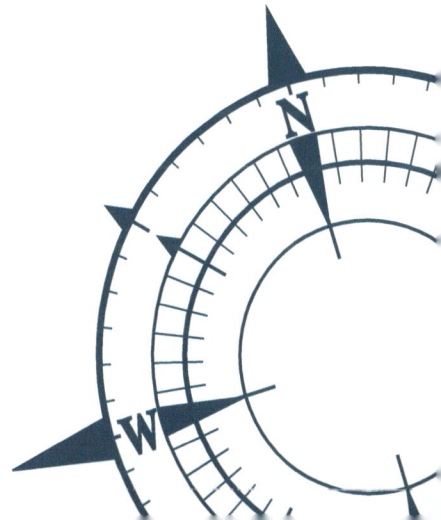

The most basic connection you

can make to the natural world

is to regain and refine

your connection to your body,

thus recognizing yourself as organic,

as a component of the ecosystem,

rather than a visitor.

The product of this synergy,

this arrival at self-awareness

is a truly holistic fitness.

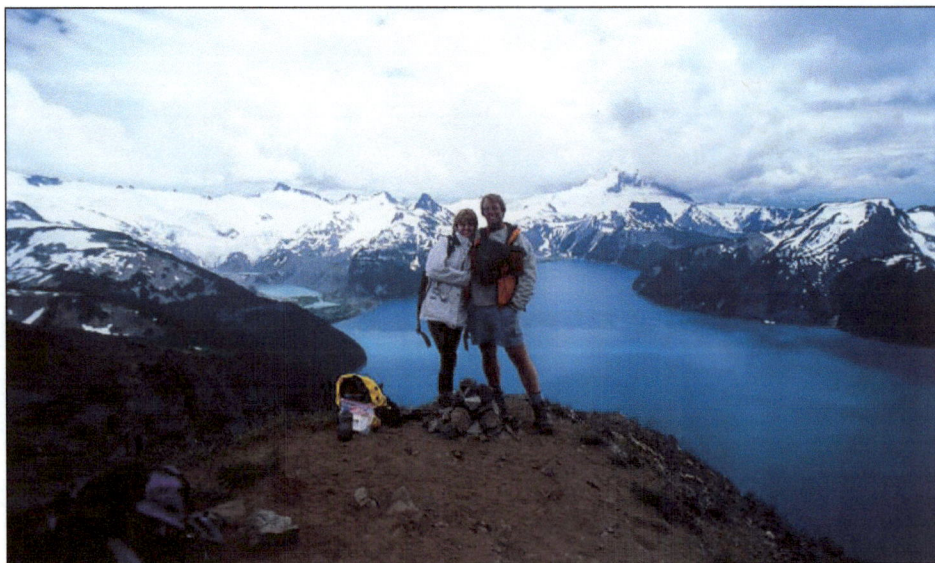

This book provides a path to a physical functionality that addresses power, endurance, core conditioning, balance and agility, flexibility and range of motion, and kinesthetic awareness through diverse, yet integrated exercises and programming that are ever-changing. This approach is specifically designed to allow you to enjoy and excel at a wide range of outdoor activities throughout the seasons of your life. Commit to yourself and to your health and you can handle whatever lies beyond the next rise in the trail, curve of the slope, or bend in the river. My intent is to help you develop the physical tools and mental confidence to get out and experience all of the beauty that nature has to offer. ***Enjoy your journey!***

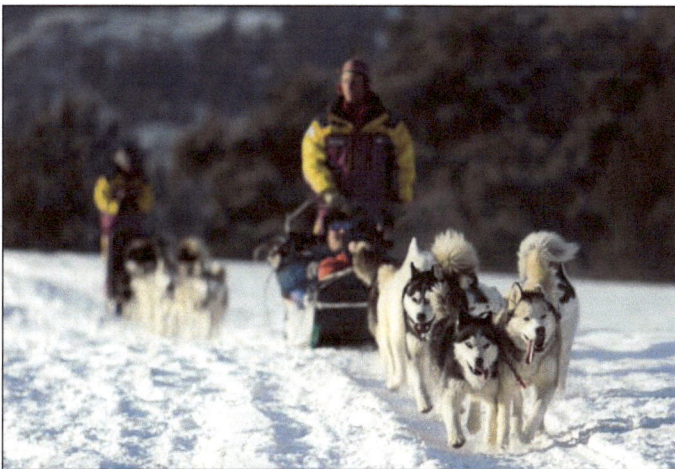

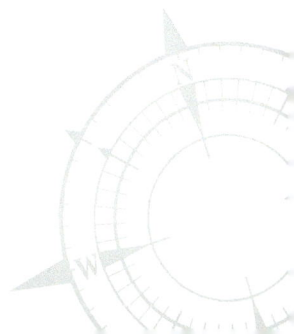

WWW.SPARTANFITNESSALASKA.COM

RESOURCES

Through time, my fitness philosophy, programming, and recreational endeavors have been shaped and improved through the insights I've gained from a multitude of resources. A few of the references on my shelf or bookmarked on my browser are listed below. Thank you to all of these individuals and organizations for the lessons they have provided and their service to fitness, outdoor recreation, and safety.

CrossFit ® is dedicated to functional fitness and affiliate gyms can be found throughout the country. They also provide programming, valuable discussion, and insightful articles in the CrossFit journal at www.crossfit.com. Further, they have developed a functional fitness program for kids. What a great concept!

Mountain Athlete (www.mtnathlete.com) offers innovative, challenging, and functional programming geared specifically for outdoor athletes. When I am looking for new ways to challenge myself and mix up my programming, I visit these two websites.

Sean Burch developed the Hyperfitness® program, which focuses on functional fitness. I often utilize his dynamic exercises in my own programming and with my clients. Sean's book Hyperfitness (Avery) and instructional DVDs are available at www.seanburch.com.

Chi Running: A Revolutionary Approach to Effortless, Injury-Free Running by Danny Dreyer and Katherine Dreyer (Fireside) and Conditioning for Outdoor Fitness by David Musnick and Mark Pierce

(Mountaineers Books) are two outstanding references for outdoor athletes.

The Mountaineers is an organization that has provided tremendous service to our community of outdoor recreationists. Its website (www.mountaineers.org) offers a wide variety of valuable information, guidance, and publications on a broad range of topics.

My longest running magazine subscription is to Outside due to its always interesting articles and valuable content (www.outside.away.com).

If you are considering working with a fitness professional, I recommend partnering with a certified personal trainer. The American Council on Exercise is one of several respected organizations with a professional certification program. You can find a listing of certified trainers in your area by visiting www.acefitness.org.

The American Red Cross offers training courses in CPR and first aid (including some courses on wilderness first aid). I recommend receiving training and staying current. For classes near you, visit www.redcross.org. Relative to first aid and survival skills, the SAS Survival Handbook: For Any Climate, in Any Situation by John "Lofty" Wiseman (Harper) is a great reference.

Snow Sense: A Guide to Evaluating Snow Avalanche Hazards by Jill A. Fredston and Doug Fesler (Alaska Mountain Safety Center) is a must if you enjoy winter recreation. Further snow and avalanche safety information can be found at www.avalanche-center.org.

The United States Geological Survey offers great resources, especially maps. Visit www.usgs.gov for more information. For orienteering basics, I recommend Staying Found: The Complete Map and Compass Handbook by June Fleming (Mountaineers Books).

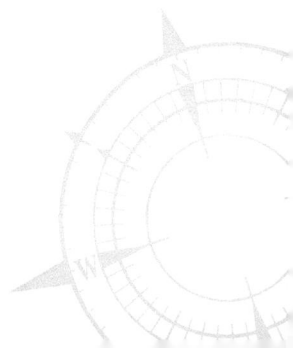

www.ingramcontent.com/pod-product-compliance
Lightning Source LLC
Chambersburg PA
CBHW060801270326
41926CB00002B/50